PreConcep

MW01243595

PreConception Miracle For Women Over 40
Improve Your Chances of Conceiving Naturally or With IVF!

A Revolutionary Holistic Approach for Women Over-40 Combining Traditional Chinese and Western Medicine to Get Your Body Ready for Pregnancy

"40 is the new 30 and getting pregnant in your 40s is the new norm."
Dr Fiona Tassoni

Dr Fiona Tassoni, MASc, BHSc
Doctor of Chinese Medicine
Fertility Coach

https://drfionatassoni.com
fiona@fionatassoni.com

Conceiving Genesis LLC
16192 Coastal Highway
Lewes, Delaware 19958 USA
+1 (302) 208-8393

Copyright Notice

IMPORTANT – PLEASE READ CAREFULLY

The User is not permitted to:

- Make print copies of the entire Book for any purpose.
- Share, rent, lease, or license the Book to any third party.
- Provide, distribute, sell, or transfer the Book or any portion thereof to any third party.
- Reproduce, translate, or modify the Book or any portion thereof.
- Distribute any electronic copy of the Book or any portion thereof on any electronic network.
- Remove or alter PreConception Miracle for Women Over 40's copyright notices, proprietary marks, disclaimers, or any other means of identification as they appear in the Book.
- By accessing, copying, printing, or otherwise using the Book, the User confirms that they have read, understood, and agree to be bound by the terms and conditions set forth in this agreement.

Book Warranty and Liability

The Book provided by the author is not guaranteed to meet the User's requirements or operate without interruption or errors. It is provided "as is" with no express or implied warranties, including but not limited to merchantability and fitness for a specific purpose. Maintenance, support, updates, enhancements, or modifications are not the obligation of PreConception Miracle for Women Over 40 or any other party involved in delivering the Book. The User assumes all risks related to the quality and performance of the Book.

PreConception Miracle for Women Over 40 will not be held liable for any damages, including incidental and consequential damages or damages for lost data or profits resulting from the use or inability to use the Book. PreConception Miracle for Women Over 40's liability is limited to the amount paid by the User for the Book license.

This license and the User's right to use the Book will be terminated if the User violates any part of the agreement. In case of termination, the User must destroy all copies of the Book.

Published by Conceiving Genesis LLC

To discuss your fertility needs, please email:
Dr Fiona Tassoni
fiona@fionatassoni.com

The information contained in this book is intended to be educational and not for diagnosis, prescription, or treatment of any disorder whatsoever.

The ideas and information offered in this book are not meant to replace the advice of a physician or other qualified health professional; they are provided with the understanding that each reader accepts full responsibility for his or her health and well-being.

This book is sold with the understanding that neither the author nor the publisher is engaged in rendering any legal, psychological,or accounting advice. Although the author and publisher disclaim personal liability, directly or indirectly, for the advice of information presented within.

Although the author and publisher have prepared this manuscript with utmost care and diligence and have made every effort to ensure the accuracyand completeness of the information contained within, they assume no responsibility for errors, inaccuracies, omissions, or inconsistencies.

Conceiving Genesis LLC
16192 Coastal Highway
Lewes, Delaware 19958 USA
(302) 208-8393
support@conceivinggenesis.com

Disclaimer

While extraordinary effort has been made to ensure the accuracy of the information in this publication, neither the Author nor the Publisher can be held accountable for any errors, omissions, or differing interpretations of the content herein. Unintentional offenses towards specific individuals, groups, or organizations are not intended.

The Author does not claim to diagnose, treat, or prevent any ailment.

This publication presents information based on the Author's personal and medical experiences and research and has not been assessed by the FDA or medical professionals.

The Author and Publisher accept no responsibility or liability on behalf of any reader or purchaser of these materials.

As with any treatment or method mentioned in this book, if in doubt, consult your physician and exercise your best judgment. Failure to do so means you are acting at your own risk.

You, as the buyer or reader of this book, assume all responsibility for any knowledge gained from this publication. Conceiving Genesis LLC and Dr Fiona Tassoni are not responsible or liable for any worsening of your condition or health issues that may arise if you discontinue medical treatment.

By choosing to utilize the information within this book, you agree to indemnify, defend, and hold harmless Conceiving Genesis LLC and Dr Fiona Tassoni from all claims (whether valid or invalid), lawsuits, judgments, proceedings, losses, damages, costs, and expenses of any kind (including reasonable attorney's fees) that Conceiving Genesis LLC and Dr Fiona Tassoni may incur as a result of using or misusing any products sold through Conceiving Genesis LLC.

Acknowledgments

1. Bensky D, Clavey S, Stöger E. Chinese Herbal Medicine: Materia Medica. Eastland Press, 2004.
2. Bensky D, Barolet R, Scheid V. Chinese Herbal Medicine: Formulas & Strategies. Eastland Press, 2009.
3. Lyttleton, J. The Treatment of Infertility with Chinese Medicine. Churchill Livingstone, 2004.
4. Deadman P, Alkhafaji M, Baker K. A Manual of Acupuncture. Eastland Press, 1998.
5. Maciocia, G. Obstetrics and Gynecology in Chinese Medicine. Churchill Livingstone, 2011.
6. Maciocia G. The Foundations of Chinese Medicine. London: Elsevier Health Sciences, 2000.
7. Maciocia G. On Blood Deficiency. EJOM;7(1):6-12.
8. Pitchford P. Healing with Whole Foods: Asian Traditions and Modern Nutrition (3rd edition). Berkeley, California: North Atlantic Books, 2002.
9. Verralls, S. Anatomy and Physiology Applied to Obstetrics. Churchill Livingstone, 1993.
10. Hadlow N, Longhurst K, McClements A, Natalwala J, Brown SJ, Matson PL. Variation in antimüllerian hormone concentration during the menstrual cycle may change the clinical classification of the ovarian response. Fertility Steril 2013:99(6):1791-1.
11. Sowers M, McConnell D, Gast K, Zheng H, Nan B, McCarthy JD et al. Anti-Müllerian hormone and inhibit B variability during normal menstrual cycles. Fertility Steril 2010;94(4):1482-6.
12. Dennis NA, Houghton, LA, Jones GT, van Rij AM, Morgan K, McLennan IS. The level of anti-Müllerian hormone correlates with vitamin D status in men and women but not boys. J Chin Endocrinol Metab 2012;97(7):2450-5.

13. Lewis R. The Infertility Cure. The Ancient Chinese Wellness Program for Getting Pregnant and Having Healthy Babies. Little, Brown, 2008.

14. Schiele F, Vincent-Viry M, Fournier B, Starck M, Siest G. Biological effects of eleven combined oral contraceptives on serum triglycerides, gamma-glutamyltransferase, alkaline phosphatase, bilirubin and other biological variables. Clin Them Lab Med 1998;36(11):871-8.

15. Calder PC, Albers R, Antoine JM, Blum S, Bourdet-Sicard R, Ferns GA et al. Inflammatory disease processes and interactions with nutrition. Br J Nutrition 2009; 101 Supps 1:S1-45.

16. Fenech M. Nutritional geonomics and the metabolic syndrome. ACMEM presentation, Adelaide May 2008.

17. Pregnancy Miracle. Lisa Olson of Higher Ways Publishing, Inc.

18. Burnham K. Alternative medicine - myasthenia gravis, Graves disease, Hashimoto hyperthyroid, Guillaine-Barre syndrome and the tiny thymus gland.

19. The Fertile Kitchen Cookbook. Cindy Bailey & Pierre Giauque, Ph.D

20. Männistö T, Vääräsmäki M, Pouta A, Hartikainen AL, Ruokonen A, Surcel HM et al. Perinatal outcome of children born to mothers with thyroid dysfunction or antibodies: a prospective population-based cohort study. Endocrine Care 2009;94(3):772-9.

21. Anand, M. The Art of Sexual Magic: Cultivating Sexual Energy to Transform Your Life. Tarcherperigee; Revised ed. edition (9 September 1996)

22. Wikland B, Sandberg PO, Wallinder H. Subchemical hypothyroidism. Lancet 2003;361(9365):1305.

23. Leggett D. Recipes for self-healing. Totnes, UK:Meridan Press 2005.

24. Barber, T. M. Why are women with polycystic ovary syndrome obese? British Medical Bulletin, Volume 143, Issue 1, September 2022, Pages 4-15.

Table of Contents

CHAPTER SIX

CHAPTER EIGHT
ENHANCING FERTILITY THROUGH LIVER DETOX: UNDERSTANDING THE BENEFITS AND EFFECTIVE TECHNIQUES

CHAPTER NINE
UNDERSTANDING YOUR HORMONAL PROFILE AND FERTILITY TESTS

CHAPTER TWELVE

CHAPTER FOURTEEN

Introduction

Dr Fiona Tassoni - Pain, Purpose, and Healing

Dr Fiona Tassoni's journey to becoming a renowned Doctor of Chinese Medicine and a global Fertility Coach began with a single, life-changing moment. It was 1997, and Fiona was a young woman working as a Legal PA at Norton Rose, one of London's largest law firms.

She was successful in her career, but something was missing. A tragic water-skiing accident at the age of 15 left her with chronic back pain, which became a daily battle for her. The pain was so excruciating that she could hardly walk, let alone live a full and happy life.

Despite years of medical treatments, nothing seemed to work for Fiona. But everything changed when she stumbled upon a Traditional Chinese Medicine (TCM) clinic on Tottenham Court Road in London. Desperate for relief, she decided to give TCM and acupuncture a try. And after just two treatments, her pain vanished, setting her on a new path.

Fiona's experience with TCM was nothing short of miraculous. It freed her from the prison of pain and ignited a passion within her to help others. She knew that she had found her calling in life and made the decision to become a Doctor of Chinese Medicine. So, she embarked on a challenging yet fulfilling journey to study this ancient healing art.

During her studies back in her native Australia, fate stepped in once more. A series of personal fertility circumstances led Fiona to discover her true passion – helping women around the world overcome fertility challenges and conceive healthy children. This newfound purpose gave her an even stronger determination to master the art of Chinese Medicine.

Dr Fiona Tassoni's mission to help women with fertility issues led her to specialize in this area of medicine. Over time, she developed a unique and highly effective approach to fertility treatment, which integrated the wisdom of Chinese Medicine with modern medical practices. As an online Fertility Coach, she dedicated her life to helping women conceive naturally before, during, or after IVF, even when their physicians had claimed it was impossible.

Her work became a beacon of hope for women all over the world, as she guided them through their fertility journey with patience, empathy, and a deep understanding of the challenges they faced. Her unwavering dedication to her patients made her one of the most sought-after fertility experts in the field.

Today, Dr Fiona Tassoni is celebrated for her extraordinary achievements in the world of fertility and Chinese Medicine. Her tireless dedication to her patients and her groundbreaking work have not only transformed the lives of countless women but also raised awareness about the importance of holistic and integrated approaches to fertility treatment.

Her story serves as an inspiring reminder that sometimes, the most powerful and life-changing experiences can arise from our deepest struggles. By following her heart and embracing her calling, Dr Fiona Tassoni transformed her pain into a life of purpose and healing, leaving a lasting legacy that will continue to inspire and empower generations to come.

PreConception and Getting Your Body Ready for Pregnancy In Your 40s

The journey to parenthood is an exciting and life-changing event for many couples. It often begins well before the pregnancy itself, with careful planning and attention to one's physical and emotional well-being. PreConception health refers to the overall wellness of an individual or couple before they conceive a child.

Emphasizing PreConception health is crucial, as it prepares the body for the incredible demands of pregnancy and ensures the best possible outcomes for both mother and child. In this book, we will explore the importance of PreConception health and discuss practical ways to prepare for a healthy pregnancy.

The Preconception Phase and its Importance

The PreConception phase, which is the 90 days leading up to conception, is crucial in determining the health of both the mother and the baby. During this period, it is essential to adopt healthy habits and make necessary lifestyle adjustments to create the best possible conditions for pregnancy. TCM offers a natural and holistic approach to achieving this balance, promoting optimal reproductive health and well-being.

Balancing Qi and Blood Flow

In TCM, the concepts of Qi (energy) and blood flow play a vital role in fertility. A balanced flow of Qi and blood within the body is believed to enhance the reproductive system's functionality, improving the chances of conception.

Acupuncture, a primary TCM technique, can be used to balance these flows by stimulating specific points in the body. This practice helps unblock any energy stagnation, promoting healthy blood flow to the reproductive organs and improving overall fertility.

Diet and Nutrients

The TCM approach to diet and nutrition focuses on the importance of nourishing the body with balanced and nutrient-rich foods. In this context, consuming specific foods can help balance the body's energy levels and improve reproductive health. For example, incorporating Kidney-nourishing foods, such as black beans and walnuts, can strengthen the reproductive system, while consuming Blood-nourishing foods, such as leafy greens and red dates, can enhance blood flow.

Chinese Herbal Medicine

Chinese Herbal Medicine, with its roots in ancient China, is a holistic healing system that has been practiced for over 3,000 years. This time-tested modality forms an integral part of Traditional Chinese Medicine (TCM), alongside acupuncture, Tui Na massage, and Qi Gong.

The philosophy behind Chinese Herbal Medicine is rooted in the principles of Yin and Yang, the Five Elements, and the interconnectedness of the human body with nature. It is believed that a balance of these forces is essential for maintaining health and well-being. When an imbalance occurs, Chinese herbalists use medicinal plants to restore harmony and promote healing.

Chinese Herbal Medicine utilizes over 6,000 plant, animal, and mineral substances in various combinations to create tailored treatments for each individual. The herbalist takes into consideration the patient's unique constitution, symptoms, and underlying imbalances to create a personalized prescription. Commonly used herbs include ginseng, astragalus, goji berries, and licorice root.

Enchancing Fertility

Preparing your body for pregnancy includes optimizing your fertility. PreConception care involves assessing and addressing any factors that could interfere with conception, such as hormonal imbalances, irregular menstrual cycles, or underlying health conditions.

Ensuring Optimal Nutrients

A well-balanced diet is essential for both prospective parents during the PreConception period. For mothers, adequate levels of key nutrients like folate, iron, and calcium can reduce the risk of birth defects and ensure proper fetal growth. For fathers, a nutritious diet can improve sperm health and increase the likelihood of a successful conception.

Strengthening Emotional and Mental Well-Being

Mental and emotional health is just as important as physical health during the PreConception period. Pregnancy and parenthood can be both rewarding and challenging, so preparing for these changes mentally and emotionally is crucial.

Addressing stress, anxiety, and depression before pregnancy can lead to a more positive experience and reduce the risk of postpartum depression.

Promoting Healthy Lifestyle Choices

Adopting a healthy lifestyle is crucial in preparing your body for pregnancy. This includes regular exercise, proper sleep, and avoiding harmful substances such as tobacco, alcohol, and illicit drugs. By making these changes before pregnancy, you can establish good habits that will benefit both you and your child throughout pregnancy and beyond.

Strengthening the Couple's Relationship

The PreConception period is an ideal time for couples to strengthen their bond and improve communication. This can help create a strong foundation for a healthy, supportive partnership during pregnancy and parenthood. Discussing your hopes, fears, and expectations can promote understanding and ensure that both partners are on the same page when it comes to family planning.

PreConception health is a vital aspect of preparing your body for pregnancy. By addressing potential risk factors, enhancing fertility, ensuring optimal nutrition, and focusing on emotional and mental well-being, you can create a strong foundation for a healthy, successful pregnancy.

Furthermore, making healthy lifestyle choices and strengthening your relationship with your partner will provide additional benefits that extend beyond conception. By prioritizing PreConception care during these 90 days, you are setting the stage for a brighter future for you and your child.

Pathway to Conception and Welcoming a Thriving Infant

For those seeking to become parents and bring a healthy child into the world, this book presents the top crucial strategies for accomplishing this naturally or with IVF. To achieve this, we need to:

- Establishing equilibrium, synergy, and alignment for welcoming your little one through a tailored approach that enhances fertility for any woman.

- Adapting your nutrition and physical activity habits to encourage conception, such as supplementing with essential vitamins and minerals, engaging in exercise, managing stress, optimizing sleep, and eliminating hazardous toxins from your environment and body.
- Revitalizing your internal organs and purifying your energy to prepare for conception using specialized acupuncture and acupressure methods designed to boost fertility.
- Guidance on harmonizing your Menstrual Cycle Phase and specific conditions using traditional Chinese herbs, in addition to incorporating fundamental Qi Gong exercises to fortify your reproductive system and unblock the necessary Qi energy channels for conception.
- Undertaking internal purification and liver detoxification to create the ideal environment for conception.

Unique Situations and Assorted Fertility Challenges

It's important to recognize that every couple's journey is distinct, resulting in varied approaches to addressing fertility concerns. We will explore some specific scenarios you might be facing, such as:

- Over 40
- Secondary fertility issues
- Tertiary infertility
- Structural infertility
- Polycystic Ovary Syndrome (PCOS), endometriosis, fibroids, and ovarian cysts
- The interplay between cancer and fertility
- Tubal ligation
- Alternative routes for couples such as IVF, yoga and massage, holistic remedies, and nurturing both physical and mental health on your path to parenthood

Some couples over 40 may prefer to read the book in its entirety before revisiting sections that address their particular concerns, while others might choose to focus on the parts that most closely relate to their situation. The way you use the information in this book is entirely up to you. Just bear in mind the significance of creating a comprehensive fertility strategy that incorporates diverse treatment techniques to maximize the likelihood of having a healthy baby.

How Doctors are Preventing Women Over-40 from Conceiving

Fertility doctors play a critical role in helping couples and individuals achieve their dream of starting a family. However, for women in their 40s, the experience of trying to conceive can be stressful and filled with fear.

This fear is often instilled by well-meaning doctors who suggest that women 40+ are too old or have old eggs or no eggs. This can create a sense of hopelessness and despair for these women, making it even more difficult for them to conceive.

It's important to understand that age is a factor when it comes to fertility, but it's not the only factor. A woman's fertility is influenced by a complex interplay of genetic, environmental, and lifestyle factors. But guess what?

... woman's fertility doesn't start and stop in her twenties. You can have a healthy pregnancy into your late 40s and beyond!

While the chances of getting pregnant naturally decrease with age, this does not mean that women 40+ can't conceive. With the right approach and support, women in their 40s can still successfully have a baby.

One of the key reasons why doctors may instil fear in women in their 40s is due to a lack of true understanding of the emotional complexity of fertility. It's true that as a woman gets older, her egg reserve decreases and the quality of her eggs declines.

However, this does NOT mean that a woman 40+ has "old eggs" or no eggs. It's important to remember that every woman is unique and there are a variety of factors that can influence a woman's fertility at any age.

Another reason why doctors may instil fear in women 40+ is due to a lack of knowledge about alternative or holistic approaches to fertility. Many doctors may only be familiar with traditional fertility treatments such as IVF and may not be aware of alternative approaches such as Chinese herbal medicine, acupuncture, or mind-body therapies.

These alternative approaches are scientifically proven to be effective in helping to improve fertility and increase the chances of a successful pregnancy.

It's important to remember that the body needs to feel safe to conceive. When the body is in a state of fear or stress, the nervous system becomes activated, releasing stress hormones that can inhibit conception.

This is why it's so important for women 40+ to work with a healthcare professional who can provide a holistic approach to fertility and who can help create a sense of safety and nourishment in the body.

When you create a sense of safety and nourishment in your body, you are allowing your body to heal, to thrive,including the cells, and the cells in your ovaries to be the healthiest that they can be and therefore you are improving your egg quality.

Chinese herbal medicine, for example, can be used to support the overall health of the reproductive system and to address specific issues that may be impacting fertility, such as hormonal imbalances, poor egg quality, and a thin endometrial lining.

Chinese herbs are chosen specifically to support the unique needs of each individual and can be used in conjunction with Western medicine to enhance the effectiveness of other treatments.

It's important for women 40+ to understand that age is a factor when it comes to fertility, but it's far from the only factor.

With the right approach and support, women in their 40s can still successfully have a baby. It's important to work with a fertility expert who understands and can provide a holistic approach to fertility using Chinese Medicine and Western Medicine.

Is the Extreme Cost of IVF in America Really Necessary if Over 40?

In vitro fertilization (IVF) is four to seven times less cost-effective for women aged 40+ than for younger women. So, finding out you have fertility problems can feel like a crushing blow.

But just as you're dealing with the pain of that, American would-be parents get sideswiped with another cruel blow, being the extremely high cost of in vitro fertilization (IVF).

The cost of IVF for each live birth in America is, on average, $38,809 for women aged 30 and under. But the average cost jumps to $107,635 for women aged 40+. Ouch!

It's often seen as the last-resort method for a woman 40+ who wants to carry her own baby, causing the demand for IVF to be higher than ever. American women are paying more for the procedure than anyone else in the world, with an average cost of around $18,000 per cycle, when you exclude the expense of medication.

However, when you factor in that additional expense, the actual cost rises to around $25,000 per cycle! With three to nine cycles generally needed to successfully result in a pregnancy, this bill can multiply fast—and that's not even including other costs like specialists' bills, co-pays, testing, and time off work.

Given these numbers, it's no wonder that only about 3% of women eligible to get IVF actually go through with it, limiting the procedure to the very wealthy or the very desperate.

Proven Cost-Cutting Solution to Getting Pregnant

Chinese medicine and a holistic approach is a scientifically proven cost-effective solution for women over 40 who are trying to conceive. Chinese medicine focuses on improving the overall health and balance of the body, including reproductive health.

By addressing any underlying imbalances or health issues, Chinese medicine can help optimize fertility and increase the chances of a successful pregnancy. Holistic approaches such as dietary changes, exercise, stress reduction techniques, and acupuncture can also support the body's natural fertility and improve overall health.

Studies have shown that acupuncture and other holistic therapies can significantly improve fertility outcomes for women 40+, while also reducing the need for expensive and invasive fertility treatments such as IVF. Overall, a combination of Chinese medicine and holistic approaches can provide a cost-effective and proven solution for women 40+ who are trying to conceive.

There are several reasons why a natural pregnancy using Chinese herbal medicine and a holistic approach can be more cost-efficient than in vitro fertilization (IVF):

① **Lower Cost:** The cost of Chinese herbal medicine and holistic therapies is generally much lower than the cost of IVF treatments. IVF can be extremely expensive and may require multiple cycles to achieve a successful pregnancy, which can add up to tens of thousands of dollars.

② **No Need for Expensive Medications:** IVF treatments often require expensive medications such as hormones and fertility drugs, which can further increase the cost of the treatment. Chinese herbal medicine and holistic approaches focus on improving the overall health and fertility of the individual, without relying on expensive medications.

③ **Fewer Risks:** IVF treatments can come with various risks and potential complications, such as ovarian hyperstimulation syndrome (OHSS), multiple pregnancies, and birth defects. Chinese herbal medicine and holistic approaches are generally safe and have fewer risks and side effects.

④ **Improved Overall Health:** Chinese herbal medicine and holistic approaches focus on improving the overall health of the individual, not just their fertility. This can lead to improved general health, increased vitality, and reduced stress levels.

⑤ **Long-Term Benefits:** Chinese herbal medicine and holistic approaches can provide long-term benefits for both the individual and the child. These approaches can help reduce the risk of future health problems, while also improving the child's overall health and well-being.

Overall, a natural pregnancy using Chinese herbal medicine and a holistic approach can be more cost-efficient than IVF, while also providing a range of additional benefits for both the individual and the child.

Why "Keep Trying" is the Worst Advice for Women Over 40!

It's a common scenario: a woman over the age of 40, who has been trying to conceive for months or even years, is told by her doctor to "keep trying."

However, as many women in this situation have found, this advice is not only unhelpful, but it can also be downright harmful. The truth is, for women 40+ who have a history of miscarriages or difficulty getting pregnant, simply "keeping trying" without addressing underlying fertility issues can lead to continued heartache and disappointment.

The good news is, there is a solution. PreConception care, or preparing your body for pregnancy over a 3-month period before attempting to conceive, can fix underlying physical and emotional fertility issues, leading to faster conception and a miscarriage-free pregnancy.

One of the most important steps in PreConception care is identifying and addressing any underlying health issues.

For example, women 40+ are more likely to have conditions such as thyroid dysfunction, polycystic ovary syndrome (PCOS), or endometriosis, which can all contribute to infertility and miscarriages.

In addition to addressing underlying health issues, PreConception care also includes lifestyle changes that can greatly improve fertility.

For example, maintaining a healthy weight, quitting smoking, avoiding alcohol consumption, and reducing stress are all important steps in preparing your body for pregnancy.

A PreConception care program may also include supplements and vitamins known to improve fertility such as Vitamin D, Vitamin B12, Folate, and iron.

Emotional well-being is also an important aspect of PreConception care. Infertility can be a very emotionally taxing experience and women who are struggling with miscarriages are likely to be dealing with feelings of grief, loss, and frustration.

A PreConception care program from a medically qualified fertility coach should include emotional support and resources to help women cope with these feelings.

It's important to note that PreConception care is not just for women 40+ who have a history of miscarriages, thyroid dysfunction, PCOS or endometriosis.

In fact, PreConception care is recommended for all women who are planning to start a family. By preparing your body for pregnancy, you increase your chances of having a healthy pregnancy and a healthy baby.

In conclusion, simply "keeping trying" without addressing underlying fertility issues is not an effective approach for women 40+ who are struggling with miscarriages and conception.

If you're 40+ and trying to conceive, or if you're planning to start a family in the near future, consider a PreConception care program to help you achieve your dream of becoming a parent.

Forward

The desire to conceive and have a child is a fundamental aspect of human nature.

However, for many women over 40, the journey to motherhood can be challenging. It can be a stressful and emotional experience, filled with disappointment and frustration.

Despite these challenges, many women over 40 have successfully conceived and given birth to healthy children.

Conception is a complex process that requires a specific set of conditions to occur. It requires a healthy reproductive system, good genes, and a favorable environment for the embryo to develop. While the technical details of reproduction are well-understood, the process itself is far more complex. Many factors can affect conception, including age, illness, genetic predisposition, and unknown barriers.

The journey to conception can be a challenging one, but it is not impossible. With the right mindset and approach, women over 40 can increase their chances of conceiving and giving birth to a healthy child. PreConception Miracle For Women Over-40 provides valuable guidance and support for women on this journey.

PreConception Miracle For Women Over-40 is not just a Book, but a comprehensive guide to help women optimize their chances of conceiving and giving birth to a healthy child. It covers everything from mindset and nutrition to lifestyle and medical interventions.

With this book as a guide, women over 40 can take control of their fertility journey and increase their chances of success.

PreConception Miracle For Women Over-40 is a must-read for any woman over 40 who is trying to conceive. It is a comprehensive guide that provides practical advice and support to help women overcome the challenges of conception and achieve their dream of motherhood.

Chapter 1

Understanding the Male and Female Reproductive Systems and the Link to Fertility

Fertility is a complex and delicate process that involves the interaction of both the male and female reproductive systems. While modern medicine has significantly advanced our understanding of these systems, traditional Chinese medicine (TCM) offers a unique and holistic approach to understanding fertility. In this book, we will delve into the basics of male and female reproductive systems and explore how TCM can shed light on fertility issues.

The male reproductive system is primarily responsible for producing and delivering sperm, while the female reproductive system is responsible for producing eggs and nurturing a fertilized egg into a developing embryo. Both systems are influenced by a complex interplay of hormones and various physiological factors, which can impact fertility.

TCM views fertility as a reflection of the overall health and well-being of both partners. The principles of TCM emphasize balance and harmony in the body, mind, and spirit, which are essential for optimal fertility.

When it comes to addressing fertility issues, TCM practitioners focus on the root causes rather than simply treating the symptoms. TCM practitioners recognize that lifestyle factors can significantly impact fertility.

They may suggest dietary changes, exercise, stress reduction techniques, and other practices to help create an environment that is conducive to conception. These recommendations are tailored to each individual's unique needs and circumstances.

TCM offers a unique and holistic perspective on fertility by focusing on the overall health and well-being of both partners. By combining acupuncture, herbal medicine, and personalized lifestyle recommendations, TCM practitioners can help address the root causes of fertility issues and support optimal reproductive health. While TCM may not be a standalone solution for everyone, it can provide valuable insights and complementary treatments for those seeking to improve their fertility.

The Female Contribution to Fertility

Women, unfortunately, have always been labeled as complicated, and this is 100% true... when it comes to a woman's reproductive organs. Let's start by looking at the science involved with how a woman is able to carry and grow a baby and how it is crucial that all aspects of her reproductive system are healthy and in the best working condition.

The Role of the Vagina

The vagina is the entry point to a woman's reproductive system and forms a natural path for the penis and sperm to pass into the womb where the sperm can undertake its most important role, fertilization.

There is one component of the vagina that can cause a potential issue when trying to get pregnant and this is the hymen. The hymen is mucosal tissue which is usually perforated with small openings and in most women, after having intercourse for the first time, the hymen is completely ripped. In a small number of individuals, the hymen can lack these perforations and as such can form a barrier stopping menstrual blood from exiting. This retrograde blood is kept in the womb and even enters into the fallopian tubes and has been shown to cause endometriosis, a common cause of infertility.

Why the Cervix is Essential

The cervix is the first essential piece of anatomy a woman needs to achieve pregnancy and remain pregnant to term. The cervix is a strong muscle-like tissue that is found at the top of the vagina prior to the womb. Its two main purposes are simple; the first is to stop infection forming in the uterus by creating a mucus barrier and the second, and arguably more important role, is to keep the baby in the womb until it is ready for delivery.

Deformities in the cervix can lead to miscarriages. Incorrect cervix formation will result in not enough resistance to keep the developing child in the womb known as an incompetent cervix. This is a relatively common deformity in women but can be overcome by stitching the opening of the cervix together until birth.

The Role of the Uterus

The normal duration of a pregnancy is around 9 months and the uterus, alternatively termed the womb, is where the baby will develop for the duration of the pregnancy.

In the past, it was commonly thought that a uterus that is retroverted (tipped back so it points towards the rectum rather than the stomach) stops women from getting pregnant however this is a myth. There are some conditions of the uterus however that can not only lead to early miscarriage but can also lead to the inability to conceive. These include:

Septate Uterus

This is a disorder that is usually formed before birth where two cavities in the womb are created due to a wall of tissue running vertically from top to bottom.

Bicornuate Uterus and Unicornuate Uterus

A bicornuate uterus is shaped irregularly and is described as a heart-shaped uterus, appearing to have two sides instead of one hollow cavity. A unicornuate uterus is a rare genetic condition in which only one-half of a girl's uterus forms. Many women who have these conditions can miscarry after conceiving.

Polyps/Fibroids

Fibroids and polyps can interfere with implantation by preventing the embryo from attaching to the uterine wall. Polyps are the endometrial outgrowths (inner lining of the uterus), while fibroids are the dense connective fibrous tissues arising from the smooth muscle of the uterus. Most polyps and fibroids can be surgically removed however this can cause excessive scarring which poses another potential problem as embryos struggle to implant on scarred areas of the uterus.

How Ovaries Play an Important Role

Having a baby naturally would be impossible without these two organs in the reproductive system. They hold all of the eggs a woman will ever have in her life as a woman already has her total egg supply at birth which is around 1 million eggs and no more are produced throughout her life.

One or two of these eggs are released every month from the ovaries to travel down the fallopian tubes for fertilization. The general life span of a released egg is 12-24 hours and if a sperm does not fertilize the egg in this time it will be removed from the woman's body during her menses. It is also known that some of the eggs in the ovaries are lost due to biological factors such as hormone imbalance. If the ovaries are subject to infection or become damaged, then this can massively impact fertility.

Why Egg Quality Matters

A healthy pregnancy is unlikely to happen without a good quantity of high-quality eggs ready for fertilization. The egg itself is the complex home of a woman's genetics which will be combined with the genetics of the sperm to dictate what the future child will look like and also will contribute to its behavioral traits too.

The human egg is not just a bubble containing genes however; it consists of three shielding layers. On the outer aspect, there is the zona pellucida or "shell", the middle layer is called the corona radiata and the final inner cumulus layer consists of cells that allow the egg to mature.

A fully developed egg, when released, is called a mature oocyte and is made up of 23 chromosomes, exactly half of how many chromosomes are required for a healthy baby. The other 23 come from the sperm which are contributed when fertilisation occurs. Should any of these chromosomes be missing, there is a high chance the baby will have an abnormality or the body will miscarry the developing child.

Healthy Fallopian Tubes are Key

As we have already discussed, one or two eggs are released on around the 14th day of a woman's menstrual cycle for fertilization. Of course, when fertilized, the egg, now an embryo, implants in the uterus to develop further however prior to this it has to make its way there. The fallopian tubes are passages that connect the ovaries to the womb and allow this journey to happen.

Healthy fallopian tubes are key for the journey of the egg from the ovary to the womb. They allow the egg to be fertilized and then move the embryo to the final destination where it will implant. As a result, even if one of your tubes has problems or blockages, it will affect your chances of becoming pregnant. For instance, a blocked tube will not allow the sperm to reach the released egg. The main conditions which can lead to damage to the fallopian tubes are infection and endometriosis.

Breaking Down the Menstrual Cycle

Between puberty and menopause, a woman will have a menstrual cycle if all her reproductive organs are performing as they should. The problem is however there are several things that can affect a woman's period but prior to discussing that let's break down the menstrual cycle into steps:

STEP 1

After bleeding has finished, a woman's pituitary gland produces follicle-stimulating hormone (FSH) in conjunction with several fluid-filled cavities, or antral follicles, in the ovaries growing to produce a mature egg.

During this follicular development, the body's estrogen production goes into overdrive and this contributes to the thickening of the uterine lining. Not only this, but the increased levels of estrogen trigger a response for more FSH and luteinizing hormone (LH) to be released.

Typically, one follicle increases in size more quickly than the others, creating more estrogen and reducing the level of FSH. This drop in hormone level stops the other follicles from growing as well as triggering the pituitary gland to create a spike in LH. This, in turn, leads to the oocyte inside the follicle becoming mature.

STEP 2

The ever-growing egg, due to maturation, eventually causes the follicle to rupture letting the egg pass into the fallopian tube. This is commonly known as ovulation.

STEP 3

If intercourse has been correctly timed, the released mature egg will encounter an enthusiastic sperm, leading to fertilization and changing the mature egg into an embryo. This embryo is then passed down the fallopian tube into the womb where it will ideally nestle into the lining and develop for the next 9 months.

STEP 4

Once released the mature egg leaves behind the outer layer of the follicle or the corpus luteum. This is important as it creates progesterone, a crucial hormone that aids the implantation process when the embryo reaches the womb lining. If the embryo doesn't stick, then the womb lining will shed and bleeding will start as part of the normal monthly menses.

After menstruation, between day 6 and day 14 of your cycle, FSH causes follicles (small sacs of fluid in your ovaries that contain a developing egg) in one ovary to begin to mature. During days 10 to 14 of your cycle, only one of the developing follicles forms a fully mature egg. Around day 14, a sudden surge of LH causes the ovary to release this egg. This is ovulation. From the start of a woman's last period, it will take these typical 10-14 days for ovulation to happen.

Time scales are incredibly important when trying to conceive. Having a longer or shorter follicular phase or cycles which are not the same length may mean your follicles are not developing when they should or in the worst-case scenario, not developing at all.

In contrast, if your luteal phase is less than 11 days which is the second phase of your cycle after ovulation, this may mean the corpus luteum is not creating enough progesterone to allow implantation.

The Importance of Timing

It is very important to know your own body for reproduction as every woman is different. Knowing your menstrual cycle and its timing will give you a better idea of when to optimally plan intercourse! The most common error in a woman's mindset is to think they are normal and just like everyone else. Thinking you are like every other woman means that you should be having sex between days 12 to 15 in your cycle as ovulation occurs on average around the 14th day, right? Well in fact, if you have been trying to conceive for a while unsuccessfully, it may be worthwhile mapping out your cycle to pin down the dates when you ovulate.

A normal menstruation cycle is 28 days long and ovulation happens roughly halfway through this, or day 14. If, however, you are noticing that your cycles are not the run-of-the-mill 28 days then your plans need to change. Let's say your periods are shorter in time apart, 25 days for instance, this would mean that ovulation will be earlier, and having sex on the 13th and 14th days will be past the window of opportunity. On the other hand, if your cycles are longer than 28 days, by the time the mature egg is released, the sperm which only has a life span of 5 days, will no longer be functioning to fertilize the egg.

To increase the probability of conception you should get planning and for most couples, it's that easy. Having sex at the optimum time of the month when you actually ovulate will make it much easier for the egg and sperm to unite.

The best time to have sex is on the day of ovulation. The most fertile days are the three days leading up to ovulation and on the day of ovulation itself however sperm can live in the reproductive tract for five days so technically, you can conceive in the five days leading up to ovulation. This is considered your fertile window and it begins five days before you ovulate. Having sex during this time gives you the best chance of getting pregnant.

However, we all know that it's not always that simple, especially if there is no set timescale for your menstrual cycle/ovulation. Having periods that are different in length on a regular basis can indicate a fertility problem. Initially, however, it is important to start understanding your body and the timings of your cycle so you have all the facts to base any future treatment.

The Male Contribution to Baby-Making

As I'm sure you are aware, making a baby is not a single-person activity! Although less complex than the female reproductive system, the male reproductive system also has come extremely important roles to play in the process of creating a baby so let's look at the anatomy of the male reproductive system and how it impacts fertility.

Why the Penis Matters

The penis is known as the "ancestral sinew" in Chinese medicine and the function of the penis is very important when considering the ability to conceive. When blood rushes to the penis and is trapped there it creates an erection. Small tubes squeeze the sperm towards the urethra and the sperm is released along with other fluids out of the penis during the process of ejaculation. If it is not possible for a male to have an erection or keep one for a certain period of time, then this is known as erectile dysfunction (ED) which can lead to difficulty conceiving.

Some research has shown a very tentative link between penis size and infertility with men with smaller penis sizes struggling to conceive however in general the medical advice is that as long as the penis is large enough to deposit the sperm up into the vagina during ejaculation then size does not matter.

The physical anatomy of the penis itself is important however and any deformity can prevent the sperm from being released in the right way to reach the egg for fertilization. Hypospadias is a very common defect in males and is where the urethra is not located in the usual central location on the head of the penis but is located elsewhere on the underside. Epispadias is a much rarer condition but is similar in that the urethra is misplaced but in this situation, it is instead on the top of the penis rather than the head.

The Sperm-Creating Testicles

Another part of the male anatomy which is important to fertility is the testicles. The testicles create and store sperm and they do this from the onset of puberty until death. The testicles are contained within a sack of skin known as the scrotum which hangs outside the body for a very important reason. For sperm and testosterone production, the testicles must be kept at a very specific temperature, 93.2 degrees Fahrenheit (34 degrees Celsius), which is 5.4 degrees Fahrenheit (3 degrees Celsius), below the normal body temperature of 98.6 degrees Fahrenheit (37 degrees Celsius).

The physical anatomy of the testicles is very important and any abnormalities can impact fertility. Common conditions include the presence of fluid or swelling around the testicle (hydrocele) or an enlargement in the veins within the scrotum (varicocele) and both conditions should be treated quickly as they can raise the testicular temperature and prevent sperm production and as a result, cause infertility.

As mentioned above, males continually produce sperm however it takes around two and a half months (74 days) for the process of mature sperm to be produced from the original germ cells. Hormones, including testosterone, LH, and FSH are involved in the process of maturation. Once matured, small tubes are known as the vas deferens squeeze the sperm towards the seminal vesicle to be combined with the seminal fluid, and then sperm moves to the urethra to be released during ejaculation.

Sperm and How Quality is on the Decline

We have learned how sperm are formed and released but how important are they in creating a baby? Well, put simply without a sperm to fertilize an egg there would be no pregnancy! Each male should have between 15 million and 200 million sperm cells per milliliter of ejaculate and therefore you will be forgiven for thinking it would be easy for just one of these to find and fertilize the egg.

However, the journey to the egg is difficult with many sperm going in the wrong direction, and therefore only around 1 million reach the fallopian tube. From there, more chemical signals should be present to help the sperm find the egg but the female environment can be particularly hostile and many are killed off before reaching the egg.

Even when a single sperm finally reaches the egg and the surface of the egg changes to ensure no other sperm enters, it takes around 24 hours for fertilization to occur.

Numerous studies have shown that there has been a decline in sperm quality in males in the past 60 years. Various factors are thought to contribute to this decline, including lifestyle changes, increased exposure to environmental pollutants and endocrine disruptors, poor nutrition, obesity, hormonal imbalance (usually testosterone), cryptorchidism (undescended testicle), alcohol, smoking cigarettes/cannabis, steroids, autoimmune diseases, sperm antibodies, mobile phones, increased stress, and other health factors.

When is the Best Time to Have Intercourse?

The correct timing of intercourse is often the key to successfully getting pregnant so proper planning is key to make sure that efforts do not go to waste!

Detecting Your Most Fertile Time

There are around 6 fertile days in every cycle when a woman is ovulating and therefore able to get pregnant when she has sex. Your "fertile window" is the five days leading up to ovulation, plus the day of ovulation. Below are a few importanttips for tracking and identifying ovulation:

Make a Calendar

Track your period dates for a few months using a diary or phone app which will give you an idea of your length of cycle and when you are likely to ovulate which is usually between cycle day 11-21.

Monitor Vaginal Fluids

During ovulation, your vaginal discharge is likely to increase and become clearer and thinner, many describe it as a raw egg white-like consistency.

Physical Changes

Other physical changes you may see or feel when ovulating are tender breasts, sharp abdomen pains, light spotting, bloating, or headaches. Your cervix will also move position lifting higher and opening slightly and therefore you can also physically check the cervix to identify ovulation.

Making Intercourse Work for You

It is not only the timing of intercourse that needs careful planning when trying to conceive. There are also some other simple tips and tricks you can use to help increase your chances of success:

- Having sex lying down and remaining laying down with your feet in the air (or against a wall) can give the sperm a little extra helping hand through gravity. For the same reasons, try to avoid going to the toilet or washing for at least 30 minutes after intercourse.

- An orgasm can help stimulate blood flow to the uterus and by stimulating the cervix after orgasm, it scoops up more semen propelling it toward the egg. If you can't orgasm through penetration then try to self-pleasure yourself after intercourse.

- There is no firm guidance as to the best sexual positions for getting pregnant so whatever is comfortable and works for you and your partner is best.

- Sperm can survive for around 5 days inside the reproductive tract so it's important to have sex in those 5 days leading up to ovulation and on the day of ovulation itself.

- The best time to have sex is on the day of ovulation so as soon as you see the LH surge in your BBT or ovulation predictor kits, you should aim to have sex within the next two days. This is when you will be at your 'peak' fertility.

The Genes to Getting Pregnant

Over the past few decades, there have been many scientific advances that have allowed us to understand more about our genetics.

Our DNA is packaged into structures found within every cell known as chromosomes. Each healthy individual will have 23 pairs of chromosomes, 46 chromosomes in total. You receive 23 from your mother and 23 from your father. They are arranged in pairs with 22 pairs being identical in males and females and 1 pair of sex chromosomes which differ, with females having an XX pair and males having an XY pair.

In a similar way, each healthy individual will have two copies of each gene, one from each parent. These genes, which are made up of DNA, are usually the same from person to person but there is variation within a small percentage of our genes which make us unique. Unfortunately, any disruption in the correct sequencing of these genes can lead to problems with pregnancy and miscarriage.

There are five main patterns through which genetic conditions can be inherited:

Autosomal Dominant – In a dominant condition, the child would only need to be given one copy of the gene, for example, the gene only needs to be passed from one parent, to cause the condition.

Autosomal Recessive – With a recessive condition, both parents need to pass on a copy of the gene for the condition to affect the child. Both parents will carry one copy of the gene, otherwise known as carriers of the condition, as they do not actively show signs of the disease. The child may have the condition, be a carrier of the condition or not inherit any copies of the gene. Statistically speaking, it is relatively rare for two carriers of a condition to find themselves together and have children, and therefore over 75% of children born with an autosomal recessive disorder are the first in their recent family line to show symptoms of the disease.

X-Linked Dominant – As discussed above, women have two X chromosomes (XX) while men only have one (XY) and for this reason, women are more likely to have an X-linked condition. As with any dominant condition, only one copy of the gene is required and therefore a mutation in the genes in only one of the X chromosomes present for a female is sufficient to cause the condition.

Males typically suffer from more severe symptoms than women with these X-linked conditions.

X-Linked Recessive – In women, the mutation must occur on both chromosomes for the condition to present itself whereas in men they can have X-linked recessive conditions with only one mutated copy of the gene. As a result, these disorders are seen more often in men than women.

Y-linked – If the mutated gene is located on the Y chromosome then it is known as a Y-linked condition. It is only possible for men to pass these conditions to their sons.

Genetic Conditions that Effect Fertility

Unfortunately, our genetic code doesn't always form perfectly and in certain individuals, their genetics contains errors that make them less likely to get pregnant or more likely to have miscarriages. Any deletions, additions, or duplications in the genetic code can lead to disease and common diseases which impact fertility are Turner Syndrome which affects women, and Klinefelter Syndrome which affects men.

As mentioned above, our DNA is packaged into structures known as chromosomes and chromosomal errors can also occur. If too many or too few chromosomes are created during embryo formation, then it is likely to cause miscarriage. Over 1 in every 500 individuals may have a translocation, where a part of the chromosome detaches and is re-attached in another location. When passed on during the fertilization process this is a major cause of repeated miscarriage.

As every year passes, science becomes more advanced, and therefore our understanding of genetics and the interaction between genetics and fertility is only increasing. Chromosomal testing (known as a Karyotype Genetic Test) can be conducted via a blood test and although it can be expensive or time-consuming, the results are invaluable for those couples finally getting an explanation as to the cause of their infertility and helping clear a path for the way forward to a successful pregnancy.

Chinese Medicine and Your Reproductive System

Chinese Medicine has been a staple in holistic health care for thousands of years, offering a low-key and non-invasive approach to addressing various health concerns. One area where it has gained increasing attention in recent years is reproductive health.

With growing interest in natural and alternative therapies, it's no surprise that many individuals are turning to Chinese Medicine to support their reproductive systems. Let's look at the key principles of Chinese Medicine and how they can benefit your reproductive health.

Foundations of Chinese Medicine

Chinese Medicine is rooted in the idea of balance and harmony within the body. It views health as a result of harmonious energy, or Qi, flowing through the body's various systems. This energy is believed to travel along pathways called meridians, which connect different organs and tissues. When Qi becomes disrupted, it can lead to various health problems, including reproductive issues.

To address these disruptions, practitioners of Chinese Medicine utilize a combination of therapies, such as acupuncture, herbal medicine, moxibustion, gua-sha, and lifestyle changes, to restore balance and harmony in the body.

Acupuncture for Reproductive Health

One of the most well-known aspects of Chinese Medicine, acupuncture involves the insertion of fine, sterile needles into specific points on the body to stimulate the flow of Qi.

Research has shown that acupuncture can be an effective treatment for various reproductive concerns, such as infertility, menstrual irregularities, and hormonal imbalances.

For instance, acupuncture has been found to improve blood flow to the reproductive organs, regulate hormone levels, improve sperm, improve egg quality, regulate your period, improve the uterine lining, increase the chances of implantation, and reduce stress — all of which can contribute to a more balanced and healthy reproductive system.

Chinese Herbal Medicine

In addition to acupuncture, Chinese Medicine also employs herbal medicine to support reproductive health. Practitioners use carefully selected herbs to create personalized formulas for each individual, addressing their unique needs and imbalances.

These herbal formulations can help regulate menstrual cycles, support fertility, and ease pregnancy-related concerns.

Chinese Medicine also emphasizes the importance of a balanced lifestyle for maintaining overall health, including reproductive health. Practitioners may recommend dietary changes, regular exercise, and stress management techniques to support a healthy reproductive system.

Additionally, self-care practices like Qi Gong and Tai Chi can help to maintain the body's energetic balance and promote overall well-being.

Lifestyle Changes and Self Care

Chinese Medicine offers a gentle and holistic approach to enhancing reproductive health. By focusing on the underlying imbalances within the body and encouraging overall harmony, it can provide a natural and non-invasive option for individuals seeking to support their reproductive systems.

Chapter 2

The Truth About Infertility When Over 40

The first thing that will cross your mind when you are actively trying for a baby with no success is that you or your partner are infertile. It is a term that we hear a lot in everyday life and media but what exactly does being infertile mean, what impact will this have on your chances of having a child and most importantly how worried do you need to be if this is the diagnosis you have just been given?

The Definition of Infertility

The definition of infertility is on the surface extremely simple, it is defined as the failure to achieve clinical pregnancy and sustain the pregnancy to full term, despite having carefully timed, unprotected sex for one year or more.

However, from this point, it gets much more complicated as couples search for a reason why they are unable to conceive. There are many different conditions or potential problems with the physical anatomy of the reproductive system which may make conceiving more difficult and a combination of these issues together may also be possible. Therefore, it can be difficult for couples to see past the diagnosis as medical professionals can struggle to identify the problem and therefore fail to see what treatment pathway is best for them either.

My aim with this book is to try and break down the barriers to infertility and explain simply the causes of infertility and possible treatments to help those currently struggling with infertility and open their minds to the different options available and ultimately have the baby that they have been dreaming of!

Potential Causes of Infertility

The diagnosis of the exact cause of infertility is extremely difficult and the severity of infertility is also wide-ranging, from couples finding it is a simple issue with timing intercourse outside of the fertile window to other couples realizing they both have physical problems with the reproductive organs that need to be corrected through major surgery.

We need to also keep in mind that infertility is only experienced by the minority, with just under 20% of couples suffering from infertility. Of all infertility cases, approximately one-third of infertility is attributed to male factors, one-third is attributed to female factors, and one-third of couples no cause can be identified, also known as idiopathic infertility.

Couples should remember that the majority of individuals are able to conceive given enough time which is why the medical professionals will always require one year of a couple actively trying before they will consider investigating further for infertility.

After this first year, if infertility is suspected, there will then be months or even years of rigorous testing to try and narrow down the list of potential causes of infertility. The exact process of testing will vary geographically but in general, it will begin with a simple questionnaire and getting a sample of the male's semen for analysis, and checking the female's pattern of ovulation to make sure they have the correct quantity and quality of sperm and eggs respectively to conceive.

Testing for Infertility

Each specialist will have their own preferred pathway for investigating infertility however there are a few tests that are commonly performed internationally.

Semen Analysis (SA)

A semen analysis is when freshly ejaculated sperm is tested in a laboratory and measured under a microscope to accurately measure the number of sperm, their motility (ability to move), their morphology (size and shape), and the volume and consistency. It is the first and most important male fertility test.

HSG (Hysterosalpingography)

An HSG is an x-ray-based test in which a liquid is injected to create a contrast to allow visualization of the anatomy of the uterus and fallopian tubes. In this way, any deformities or blockages can be easily seen and steps can be taken to correct the issue to increase the chance of pregnancy.

Laparoscopy

This procedure involves the use of a camera which is inserted through the wall of the abdomen to examine any organs in the surrounding area but in the case of infertility the uterus, fallopian tubes, and ovaries are of particular importance. Physical deformity or another disease may be visualized in this way.

Conditions Affecting Fertility

There are a number of different conditions which are routinely diagnosed and may be determined to be a contributing factor to your infertility. These include:

Insufficient Nutrients

If the diet is poor and the patient is either under or overweight then this can impact fertility.

Disorders of the Endocrine

The endocrine system is a complex process involving chemical messengers and hormones. Problems with parts of the endocrine system such as the thyroid, pituitary gland, or adrenal gland can cause problems with conceiving.

Autoimmune Thyroid Disease

Hashimoto's Thyroiditis which presents with symptoms of an underactive thyroid (Hypothyroidism) and Grave's disease, which presents with symptoms of an overactive thyroid (Hyperthyroidism).

Disorders of the Vagina

A hymen that hasn't been perforated correctly can cause infertility along with physical issues such as a shorter or narrower vagina (known as stenosis) which can all impact on correct physical penetration of the penis. Inflammation of the vagina, known as vaginitis can also damage sperm in some cases.

Disorders of the Cervix

Inflammation is also possible in the cervix, usually as a result of a sexually transmitted infection and this is known as cervicitis. Polyps can also grow causing blockages and preventing the travel of sperm.

Disorders of the Uterus

The surface or shape of the uterus can be deformed and in this instance, the embryo will not be able to correctly implant.

Disorders of the Ovaries

Abnormalities in the ovaries can be present from birth or develop at a later age and any cysts or other deformity can prevent normal ovarian function and as a result cause or contribute to infertility.

Tube Blockage

It is very common for women suffering from infertility to suffer from blocked fallopian tubes. Fertilization is nearly impossible in this situation as the sperm and egg have very little chance of meeting.

PCOS

Polycystic Ovary Syndrome (PCOS) is a hormonal and metabolic disorder, that affects ovulation which means there can be no periods, or periods that are irregular or infrequent causing fertility problems.

Age-Related Factors

Women over the age of 40 years old may find their egg quality or egg quantity declining rapidly.

Emotional Factors

Chronic stress can alter hormone levels, potentially affecting fertility in both men and women. Anxiety and depression can also have indirect effects on fertility; they may lead to sexual dysfuntion and irregular menstrual cycles.

External Factors

Couples often do not realize that products such as feminine hygiene products or lubricants can alter the natural environment of the vagina, by increasing acidity which in turn can damage sperm when it enters the vagina.

Male-Related Issues

Although less complex than the female reproductive system, there are also a few issues related solely to men which should be considered including the volume, shape of the sperm (morphology), number of sperm (concentration/count), and the movement of the sperm (motility).

The Hostile Uterus

The first condition we will consider in depth is that of the hostile uterus which is an extremely common problem among infertile women. When the hormones are imbalanced, it will create a hostile environment for the sperm causing damage or destroying the sperm completely on its journey to the fallopian tubes to meet with and fertilize the egg.

A hostile uterus can be caused by different conditions including hormonal changes, a higher-than-normal level of anti-sperm antibodies, or infection.

Tests to detect a hostile uterus may include examining for any changes in the mucus, inflammation, or infection. Additionally, post-coital testing is commonly performed 8-12 hours after intercourse to check the motility or movement of the live sperm to determine if the sperm stays viable after sexual intercourse and contact with the mucus. Doctors inspect the behavior of the sperm in the cervical mucus and assess its quantity and quality (stretching and color).

There are several treatment options depending on the exact cause of the hostile environment:

• Treating any infection or inflammation present using antibiotics.

• Treating any changes in the mucus using hormone replacement medication such as estrogen tablets.

• If the problem is immune-related, such as the presence of too many anti-sperm antibodies, steroids may be given although this is usually a last resort as the side effects of the medication can be severe.

• The final 'treatment' is the most effective and that is to completely avoid the hostile environment through the use of in vitro fertilization (IVF) or intrauterine insemination (IUI).

Male Infertility

We have identified a number of female-related fertility problems but let's briefly consider those issues which males may face when trying to conceive. Male problems account for one-third of all cases of infertility experienced by a couple and therefore it is important to understand the potential fertility problems which males experience too.

The most important part of the male reproductive system is the sperm and therefore there are understandably a few common issues related to the sperm. Where a male has no sperm at all then this is known as azoospermia and this will result in complete infertility.

Similarly, a male may have a low volume of sperm (less than 15 million sperm/mL), known as oligospermia, and in this instance conceiving is possible but will be much more difficult.

Where there is a complete lack of sperm, or the sperm is of extremely poor quality, a sperm donor will be required however there are a few treatments that may help increase the production of sperm such as hormonal supplements.

Another sperm-related condition commonly faced by men is retrograde ejaculation and, in this instance, the semen will not exit through the penis during ejaculation but instead ends up in the bladder and as a result, fertilization will not be possible as the sperm remains in the male, and is not ejaculated into the female to reach the egg.

The final condition we will consider is hypospadias, a congenital condition in which the penis does not develop correctly and the urethra is in the incorrect place causing infertility through associated testes problems.

As the age of first-time fathers continues to rise, it is important to address the issue of male infertility, especially for men over 40. Aging not only affects women's fertility but can also have a significant impact on men's reproductive health.

Causes of Male Infertility Over 40

① **Age-related decline in sperm quality:** As men age, the quality of their sperm tends to decline. This can include lower sperm count, reduced sperm motility, and an increased percentage of abnormally shaped sperm. These factors can make it more difficult for the sperm to fertilize an egg, resulting in reduced fertility.

② **Varicocele:** A varicocele is an enlargement of the veins within the scrotum, which can cause a decrease in sperm quality. Varicoceles are more common in older men and can be a contributing factor to infertility.

③ **Lifestyle factors:** Poor lifestyle choices such as smoking, excessive alcohol consumption, and obesity can all negatively impact male fertility. These factors can lead to hormonal imbalances and decreased sperm production, making it harder to conceive.

④ **Medical conditions:** Certain medical conditions, like diabetes, can affect male fertility by causing nerve damage and impairing blood flow to the reproductive organs. Additionally, some medications used to treat chronic conditions can also have a negative impact on fertility.

Solutions for Male Infertility Over 40

Male infertility is often linked to factors such as low sperm count, poor sperm motility, and abnormal sperm morphology. Age plays a crucial role in male fertility, as the quality and quantity of sperm production decline with time. Men over 40 may face issues such as DNA fragmentation, hormonal imbalances, and oxidative stress, which can contribute to infertility.

Traditional Chinese Medicine's Approach to Male Infertility

TCM has a long history of treating male infertility using a holistic approach that focuses on balancing the body's energy or "Qi." This is achieved through a combination of herbal remedies, acupuncture, dietary adjustments, and lifestyle changes. The primary goal of TCM is to address the root cause of infertility by enhancing overall health and well-being.

① **Herbal remedies:** TCM utilizes various herbal formulations to improve sperm production, quality, and motility. These herbs have anti-inflammatory, antioxidant, and hormone-regulating properties that help restore balance to the reproductive system. Some popular herbs used in treating male infertility include Ginseng (Ren Shen), Astragalus (Huang Qi), Cuscuta (Tu Si Zi), and Epimedium (Yin Yang Huo).

② **Acupuncture:** Acupuncture is another cornerstone of TCM, involving the insertion of thin needles at specific points on the body to stimulate energy flow. Acupuncture has been shown to increase blood flow to the reproductive organs, reduce inflammation, and regulate hormonal imbalances. Studies have indicated that acupuncture can improve sperm quality and increase the chances of successful conception.

③ **Dietary and lifestyle changes:** TCM practitioners also recommend dietary modifications and lifestyle adjustments to promote fertility. Consuming a balanced diet rich in antioxidants, vitamins, and minerals is essential to support sperm health. Reducing stress, getting adequate sleep, and engaging in regular exercise can also improve overall health and fertility.

Traditional Chinese medicine offers a promising alternative for men over 40 experiencing infertility. By focusing on the root causes and addressing the body's overall health, TCM provides a comprehensive approach to improving fertility.

Female Infertility

Thinking again about the female reproductive system there are a few other conditions that we have yet to explore.

Anovulation

When an egg isn't released by the ovaries during the cycle it is known as anovulation. Typical causes are:
• Mental conditions such as depression, anxiety, or stress
• Physical conditions such as diabetes, anemia, tuberculosis, or inflammatory bowel disease
• A diet of insufficient nutrients or anorexia
• Over-exercising or lack of sufficient rest
• Imbalance in hormone levels
• Prescribed medication or the use of recreational drugs
• Conditions of the ovaries or pituitary gland

Damage to the Fallopian Tubes

The fallopian tubes connect the uterus and the ovaries and are where conception happens therefore blockage or damage to the tubes will result in infertility.

Treatment to rectify blockage or damage includes surgery to unblock the tube/s, remove scar tissue, repair tissue damage, or reverse previous tubal ligation surgery where tubes are cut or tied. Another treatment can be IVF where the follicles are removed and fertilized out with the body and then the embryo is placed back directly into the uterus.

Miscarriage/Pregnancy Loss

The term miscarriage refers to any spontaneous abortion or pregnancy loss before 24 weeks. Two or more pregnancy losses are defined as recurrent miscarriage or recurrent pregnancy loss (RPL).

As mentioned above, early pregnancy loss is extremely common with more than 50% of all pregnancies ending this way and therefore suffering from a miscarriage does not automatically mean you are infertile. It is only when you have suffered several miscarriages that your specialist will consider that there is a bigger issue that may be causing the pregnancy to be lost before full term.

Some of the most likely causes of pregnancy loss are as follows:

Genetic Abnormalities

Abnormalities can occur in the genetics of either the embryo or the parents themselves. In the embryo/fetus, chromosomal errors can occur during the recombination of the DNA from the mother and father and this is in fact a very common occurrence, with over 70% of miscarriages being a result of a fetal chromosomal error. It is also possible that the parents can suffer from a genetic abnormality which means they are more likely to suffer from miscarriage and this can be passed down the genetic line.

Autoimmune Issues

Autoimmune issues involve the body incorrectly targeting and damaging its own cells and autoimmune disease can be a common cause of miscarriage.

Physical Abnormalities

Incorrect physical formation or deformity in any part of the reproductive system, but particularly the uterus can cause miscarriage.

Disease

Many diseases make it more difficult to conceive and in a similar way diseases such as diabetes and thyroid problems also make it difficult to sustain pregnancy to term.

Environmental Issues

There are many man-made and naturally occurring substances that are known to cause miscarriage. These include drugs, medications, nicotine, alcohol, cleaning products, caffeine, and anesthetics among many others therefore pregnant women must be extremely careful to only consume safe substances and be conscious of their environment to avoid miscarriage.

Understanding Female Infertility Over 40

Female infertility can be influenced by various factors, including age, medical conditions, and lifestyle choices. In women over 40, the most common cause of infertility is the decline in egg quality and quantity. This natural process, known as ovarian aging, results in fewer available eggs and a higher likelihood of chromosomal abnormalities. Consequently, women over 40 often face more significant challenges in conceiving, maintaining a healthy pregnancy, and delivering a healthy baby.

Reading Your Body – When Are You Most Fertile

Finding your fertile window is one of the simplest but most important first steps to take if you are struggling to conceive. You can only conceive when you are ovulating so learning to identify your body's ovulation signals is the easiest thing you can do to help yourself on the path to getting pregnant. Let's take a look at the different changes that occur as you ovulate and how you can identify them.

Identifying Cervical Mucus Changes

As a woman, you will always have vaginal discharge but the subtle changes in texture can be easily overlooked unless you know what you are looking for.

Throughout your menstrual cycle, the mucus produced by the cervix will change in consistency and volume depending on whether you are ovulating or not.

Your mucus becomes clearer, wetter, and more viscous at the time of ovulation so these are the initial signs to be aware of. The various stages of your cycle and the impact this has on your discharge are given below:

Infertile Phase

In every cycle you will have a period where you are infertile and won't conceive, during this time you will experience very little cervical mucus or discharge.

Fertile Phase

Approaching ovulation, the quantity of mucus will increase and you may begin to notice it more. It will still be creamy-colored at this stage in your cycle and will be moist and almost sticky to the touch.

As we continue in the cycle toward your peak fertile window, the mucus will continue to increase in volume and become stretchier and cloudy-colored.

As you get closer to ovulation, and your estrogen levels increase, the mucus will continue to grow in volume and will get thinner and clearer resembling a raw egg white. The mucosal changes at this time of the cycle are designed to support the sperm to survive and reach the egg safely once released.

The Fertile Window

On the final fertile day of your cycle, you will notice the thinner, more transparent discharge which is a clear consistency that is slippery and very wet and after this point, it will begin to change as your fertile window passes. This day is usually the exact day or within a few days of ovulation.

Needless to say, this is the optimum time of your cycle to have intercourse as it is the time you are most likely to achieve pregnancy. The mucus is most fertile at this stage to ensure sperm live and travel safely to the egg upon ovulation ready for fertilization to take place.

Post-Ovulation

Your mucus will reduce in volume and become drier after the fertile window due to hormonal changes. Higher progesterone levels will cause the mucus to thicken in order to stop sperm from entering the cervix at the incorrect time of the month.

Checking Your Cervical Mucus

It is extremely easy to check your mucus, you just need to know what to feel and look for. While on the toilet you can use your finger to feel the mucus in the central mouth of the vagina, not the walls.

You will also have vaginal fluids so you need to make sure you are feeling and testing the cervical mucus itself. An easy way to identify the fluid is to place it into a cup of water. If it sinks it is cervical mucus but if it dissolves into the water it is normal vaginal fluid and not helpful for determining ovulation. Cervical mucus is insoluble.

How to Feel Mucosal Changes

You may still be struggling to tell if the mucus you are feeling is particularly wet or dry, stretchy or not so here are some helpful hints to guide you:

- **Dry:** Imagine placing your lips on your arm and the dry feeling as you rub them along your skin.

- **Wet:** Now imagine the difference if your lips or arm were wet from saliva before you rub them and this is what a wetter mucus will feel like.

- **Slippery:** Finally, at your most fertile time your mucus will be very wet slippery. Imagine putting on lip gloss and then rubbing your tongue over your lips. This lack of friction is what you expect from your mucus at your most fertile time of the month.

BBT Temperature

Basal body temperature (BBT) is likely something that you are vaguely aware of, regardless of how long you have been trying to conceive. Knowing when to have intercourse to become pregnant will obviously give you a greater chance of it actually happening, not to mention if you are struggling to conceive it can also identify more serious conditions such as a luteal phase defect.

Do you understand what BBT actually is though or how to measure it? Put simply, it is your body temperature at rest. It is essential to get an accurate reading which means the temperature should be taken as soon as you wake. Yes, this means taking a reading before doing your usual morning routine; getting out of bed, making a cup of tea, and your usual bathroom habits. Taking your temperature is relatively simple. All you need is a digital thermometer that will decipher your temperature to 0.1 of a degree, making it easier to record your BBT and its subtle changes.

Recording your temperature at the same time every day means you will soon see the fluctuations during your cycle which will give you a good indication of when you will ovulate. It is of course essential that the temperature is observed at a consistent time each day and it is also important to note that the temperature can be affected by inconsistent sleep patterns. Ideally, you're looking for 3 hours of interrupted sleep before you take the temperature.

It is of course natural that your BBT will go up and down on a daily basis, generally by 0.1 of a degree. You can guarantee that if you see a spike where the temperature goes up 0.2 degrees and stays consistently elevated for 3 consecutive days, you will have ovulated. Recording your temperature is an investment in time, however, as you will only be able to estimate when you ovulate after many months of gathering the temperatures on a daily basis. Regular readings will allow you to understand your BBT changes and see if you are releasing an egg. If your temperature doesn't change in the expected way throughout the month then this is when you should be seeking medical advice.

Recording Your Body Temperature

So, you're now up to speed on what your basal body temperature is and the importance of it but how to take it easily and make sure you are giving yourself the most accurate result. Some handy hints are:

- Purchase a digital thermometer.
- Start recording on Day 1 of your cycle and always begin marking a new chart on Day 1 of your period.
- Measure your temperature as soon as your eyes open and before getting up out of bed.
- Track your temperature on a chart or app and be sure to comment if you have any issues with your temperature for instance having a fever or poor deep quality. Also, note when you have intercourse with the letter "I" and use symbols to describe your cervical mucus changes.
- Use S (for sticky), SCM (for sticky cervical mucus), C (creamy), or CCM (creamy cervical mucus), D (dry), W (watery), WCM (watery cervical mucus), EW (egg white), EWCM (egg white cervical mucus).
- During your period, you can mark your period with a B (for bleeding) or M (for menstruation).

Why Does the Temperature Rise?

When you ovulate your progesterone hormone levels rise and this is what causes an increase in body temperature. It is impossible for your BBT to increase if ovulation doesn't happen, so make sure to stay alert for extended periods of higher temperature.

There are different ways that a BBT can change, below are some of the frequent patterns to look out for when charting your recordings:

- **Sloping Increase** – It is important to understand your body temperature doesn't need to jump to a higher reading on the day of ovulation. A slow elevation, normally displayed as an arc, over a few days will also indicate ovulation.

- **Slow Increase** - Nearly the same as the first mentioned scenario, a balanced slow rise of 0.1 degrees over the period of a few days can also indicate ovulation.

- **Fallback Increase** – This is a more aggressive pattern that shows a sharp elevation of temperature initially. A subsequent dip is then seen leading to a higher steadier temperature during the luteal phase of your cycle.

- **Staircase Increase** - As the name suggests, in this scenario your temperature increase stays consistent, or even reduces, and then increases back to a constant reading until a higher reading is eventually seen.

Determining pregnancy is usually completed by observing 3 distinct temperatures. Pre-ovulation, ovulation, and post-ovulation temperatures which is known as a triphasic chart. When you get this pattern on your BBT chart, you can almost be certain there will be a positive result after doing a pregnancy test!

Cervical Assessment

Temperature is not the only factor that can be considered when trying to identify if you are ovulating. The cervix can also feel different at different times during your cycle and knowing the differences can help you determine the best time to have sex. If the cervix is difficult to palpate and is more moist than usual this can indicate ovulation as the cervix will retract back into the uterus, opening it slightly and allowing sperm to enter. On the contrary, if your cervix is drier and harder this would indicate that you are not ovulating and the cervix would most likely be closed.

Examining Your Cervix

This isn't hard and you don't need a doctor to help, you can do it all by yourself. It is however important to know what you are feeling and make sure you use well-washed hands; you don't need to be fully sterile but you do need to be clean.

Initially, try to identify how hard the cervix is. As mentioned above, when the cervix becomes softer it is letting you know that ovulation is happening and it is the best time to be having sex if trying to conceive. Knowing the orientation of the cervix comes second. A higher cervix, in some cases an inch higher, will indicate ovulation which will gradually lower after this has happened. The final thing to identify is if your cervix is open or closed. If you can put your finger into the opening this indicates ovulation allowing sperm to pass through to find the newly released egg.

Being in a consistent posture, usually having a single foot on a low footrest will help. Pass your finger into the vagina all the way until you feel the back. This is where you will feel your cervix, usually on the end of the finger. If you are having trouble, try putting pressure on your abdomen. If you do need to do this however make sure you do the same thing every time, regularity is key when documenting your findings.

It is really important that you do not compress the cervix. Instead when investigating whether it is open or closed as well as the position and hardness, gently use your finger to remove any mucus in the area. Then take your finger out and examine the mucus utilizing what was suggested previously.

When to Leave Your Cervix Alone

The main time you should leave your cervix alone is when menstruating. You won't feel anything important or useful related to your fertility now and can also pass on infections.

Additional times when you shouldn't be checking are:

• Just after waking up, the cervix is generally higher and can lead to a false reading.
• After defecation, this can change the orientation of the cervix.
• During an STI, specifically genital warts or herpes.
• After discovering abnormal Pap smear test results, don't check until you are cleared.

Creating a Cervical Timeline

As I've already mentioned, the best time to have sex if you are trying to get pregnant is when your cervix is higher, less firm, and open. This time is generally labeled as your peak day and is the final day of any fertile signs.

We have talked a lot about knowing what a fertile cervix feels like but it is important to know what the opposite feels like as well. You won't get a good idea about this and when changes to your fertility are happening until your findings have been tracked for a few cycles.

The most straightforward way of recording your findings is on a chart or app. If your cervix is closed, then put a dot on your chart/app and if it is open draw a circle or use the symbol "O" for open.

The same goes for illustrating if your cervix is high or low on your chart, make sure you mark it clearly and consistently with your findings and drawings. Don't forget to add comments about anything you cannot draw, for instance, how hard your cervix is or the consistency of the mucus.

The Importance of Hormones

If you ask any woman, they will tell you that their body is governed by hormones. Even more so when attempting to get pregnant. If there is a discrepancy in any one of a woman's hormones during a cycle, then there is a very slim chance that she will even conceive let alone develop and grow a baby for 9 months.

About Reproductive Hormones

For example, LH and FSH tell your ovaries when to release eggs. Other hormones, such as progesterone and prolactin, also play a role in fertility. When these hormones are out of balance, ovulation may occur less often or not at all. You may experience irregular ovulation.

A woman's fertility can also be impacted by imbalances in hormones due to other factors, such as:

• Polycystic ovary syndrome (PCOS)
• Overactive or underactive thyroid
• Conditions that cause the release of excess stress hormones
• Reduced levels of estrogen, the female sex hormone

A man's hormone levels can also affect his ability to impregnate his partner. FSH, LH, and testosterone are the three main hormones that drive male fertility. LH primarily stimulates testosterone production, while FSH stimulates the production of sperm. The testes must be capable of responding to this hormonal stimulus.

The Importance of Spermatozoa

Creating a baby is impossible without healthy sperm. Your partner at the end of the day only needs one healthy sperm to fertilize a woman's egg but if you are struggling to get pregnant, then determining the quality of your partner's sperm via semen analysis is suggested.

A semen analysis (SA) is the first and most important male fertility test. It accurately measures the number of sperm, their motility (ability to move), their morphology (size and shape), and the volume and consistency of the ejaculated sample.

It's as simple as requesting a test form and booking an appointment. Your Fertility Specialist or doctor can provide a request form for a semen analysis. You will be required to produce a semen sample by masturbation, after at least three days of abstinence from sexual activity.

You collect the entire ejaculated amount in a clean, dry container which is provided by your Fertility Specialist or doctor.

Some clinics have a private room to collect the sample or you can produce a sample at home and bring it to the collection center or clinic within one hour.

The initial observation will be how the sperm looks and if it can be categorized as "normal". Sperm is made up of 3 parts, the head, neck or midpiece, and the tail and there are several common issues that are typically identified.

Sperm Head Development

All of the genes being passed on by the father are stored in the sperm head. A head that is overly large, spherical, or even if there are two heads will inhibit correct fertilization of the egg.

Sperm Movement

As already mentioned, fertilization happens in the fallopian tubes. In order for the sperm to get there they need sufficient energy to make the journey. This is provided by fructose and if there is a lack of this the sperm simply won't get to the egg.

Sperm Tail

Having sperm without a tail, more than one tail, or coiled tails will stop it from swimming properly and as such will stop it from reaching the egg to fertilize it.

There is a benchmark of what "normal" sperm should resemble and this has been determined by the World Health Organisation (WHO). In order for your partner to have normal sperm which can create a pregnancy, it needs to fall into the following parameters:

• **Volume** - Roughly a teaspoon or between 1.5ml to 5ml should be produced
• **Concentration** - Per sample, there should be a sperm count ranging from 15 million sperm to more than 200 million per milliliter (mL) of semen. Anything less than 15 million sperm per milliliter is considered low.
• **Motility** - A greater number than 40% should be seen moving in the sample.
• **Morphology** - This is how the sperm look and more than 4% of the sperm should look normal. The reference range is 4-48%. Anything less than 4%, unfortunately, means your partner's fertility is poor.

There are additionally more in-depth measurements such as:

• **Forward progression of sperm** - This is a scale from 1-4 and anything lower than 2+ means your sperm is not swimming optimally.

• **White blood cells** - There shouldn't be more than 5 per area seen under the microscope.

• **Hyper-viscosity** - Coagulation should happen soon after ejaculation followed by liquefying after around 20 minutes.

• **pH level** – The environment needs to be alkaline to inhibit the effects of vaginal acid.

• **Hypo-Osmotic swelling test** - When brought into contact with a hypo-osmotic solution at least 50% of the sperm should swell showing normal function.

• **Anti-sperm antibodies** - If these are present they can affect how the sperm swim as they attach to the tail and prevent correct function.

• **Acrosome reaction test** - In order to penetrate the egg, the sperm head needs to have a dual layer of enzymes named the acrosome. A lack of this layer leads to the diagnosis of infertility.

Quality Over Quantity Sex: The Key to Conceiving Over 40

When you're over 40 and trying to conceive, the focus on quality sex becomes even more important. Many couples in their 40s face unique challenges in their journey to parenthood, including age-related fertility declines and increased risks of complications.

To maximize your chances of conceiving, it's essential to prioritize good quality sex, which not only helps improve the likelihood of pregnancy but also strengthens the emotional bond between partners.

The Importance of Good Quality Sex When Trying to Conceive Over 40

① **Emotional Connection:** Fostering a strong emotional bond between partners is vital for couples trying to conceive. Good quality sex helps strengthen this bond, providing a foundation of trust, intimacy, and love that can make the conception journey more enjoyable and less stressful.

② **Hormonal Balance:** Engaging in satisfying, pleasurable sex can help balance hormones such as oxytocin, serotonin, and dopamine. These hormones not only enhance mood and promote relaxation but also play a role in regulating menstrual cycles and improving overall reproductive health.

③ **Improved Sperm Quality:** For men over 40, sperm quality may decline due to factors such as age, stress, and environmental toxins. Good quality sex, characterized by deep arousal and orgasm, can lead to healthier sperm, increasing the chances of conception.

Chapter 3

The Unison of Traditional Chinese Medicine and Western Medicine for Women Over 40

Examining Fertility: The Differences Between Eastern and Western Medicine and How to Increase Your Chances of Getting Pregnant

For couples trying to conceive, the journey to parenthood can sometimes prove to be a challenging one. With numerous treatment options available, it's essential to understand the differences between Eastern and Western medicine to make informed decisions that can increase your chances of getting pregnant.

Eastern Medicine: A Holistic Approach to Fertility

Eastern medicine, with its roots in Traditional Chinese Medicine (TCM), emphasizes a holistic approach to fertility. It aims to achieve balance within the body, addressing not just the physical aspects but also the emotional, mental, and spiritual aspects of a person's health.

Key components of Eastern medicine for fertility include acupuncture, herbal medicine, and lifestyle modifications.

① **Acupuncture:** This ancient Chinese practice involves inserting fine needles into specific points on the body to balance the flow of energy or Qi. Research suggests that acupuncture can help improve blood flow to the reproductive organs, regulate hormones, and reduce stress – all factors that can contribute to improved fertility.

② **Herbal Medicine:** Eastern medicine practitioners often prescribe customized herbal formulas to address various fertility issues. These formulas can help regulate menstrual cycles, support ovulation, and improve the overall health of the reproductive system.

③ **Lifestyle Modifications:** Eastern medicine also emphasizes the importance of a balanced lifestyle, including proper nutrition, exercise, and stress reduction techniques like meditation, Tai Chi and Qi Gong. These practices are believed to create a nurturing environment for conception.

Western Medicine: Targeted Intervention for Fertility

In contrast, Western medicine focuses on targeted interventions and uses advanced diagnostic tools to identify specific fertility issues. Treatment options in Western medicine include medications, assisted reproductive technologies (ART), and surgical procedures.

① **Medications:** Fertility drugs, such as Clomid or gonadotropins, are often prescribed to stimulate ovulation and improve the chances of conception. These medications regulate or induce ovulation, increasing the likelihood of successful fertilization.

② **Assisted Reproductive Technologies (ART):** In vitro fertilization (IVF) and intrauterine insemination (IUI) are common ART procedures. These treatments involve the direct manipulation of eggs and sperm to increase the chances of successful fertilization and implantation.

③ **Surgical Procedures:** When structural abnormalities or blockages in the reproductive system are identified, surgical intervention may be necessary. Procedures such as laparoscopy or hysteroscopy can help remove obstructions or repair issues that may be hindering conception.

Integrating Eastern and Western Medicine for Optimal Fertility

For couples struggling with infertility, a combined approach that incorporates both Eastern and Western medicine may offer the best chance for success. By addressing the underlying causes of fertility issues, such as hormonal imbalances and stress, Eastern medicine can provide a solid foundation for the targeted interventions of Western medicine.

For example, acupuncture and herbal medicine may be used to optimize the body's overall health and prepare it for fertility treatments such as IVF or IUI. At the same time, lifestyle modifications can help reduce stress and create a supportive environment for conception.

Understanding the differences between Eastern and Western medicine is crucial when exploring fertility treatment options. While Eastern medicine focuses on achieving balance and overall well-being, Western medicine targets specific fertility issues with advanced diagnostics and interventions. By combining the strengths of both approaches, couples can increase their chances of achieving a successful pregnancy and ultimately, parenthood.

Questioning the Existence of Infertility

Not being able to conceive can be a result of more factors than you care to imagine, however, being told outright that you cannot have a child at all is unfair, especially if a female's reproductive organs are not defective. Unless there is a complete failure of the reproductive organs such as a complete physical deformity, pregnancy is always a possibility and, although sometimes harder than usual, it can be achieved with adequate support and time invested into the diagnosis and treatment.

In today's world, it can be easy to spend a lot of money on seeking the best medical technology and specialists involved in modern science to try to get an answer as to why getting pregnant is proving difficult. Dwelling solely on these practices, however, is not the only way you can improve your chances of conceiving. Thankfully there are several natural options within Chinese medicine that couples all over the world have been using extremely successfully to improve their fertility.

If you have been on the road to conceiving and have been constantly encountering setbacks that slow the process down, there is no better time to investigate every option available to you. The fortunate thing is that many readers who pick up this book will be able to conceive, it's simply a case of determining how Eastern medicine in particular can help to determine the specific path to success that is right for you.

The opinions and treatment options of Eastern and Western medicine are varied so let's now look into these approaches in more detail and see how you can help to improve your chances of having a baby.

The Eastern Perspective on Fertility

The basic foundation of the Eastern approach to medicine is that each health issue, fertility included, is influenced by a person's connection to their environment. As I will go on to discuss, causality is the backbone of Eastern medicine and this is never more apparent than in the relationship between the environment and your health.

In Chinese culture, the belief is that the human entity is a complicated ecosphere and even the most minute change can put everything else out of balance. In Traditional Chinese medicine, no single aspect of a human will be left ignored and the connection between all aspects is always considered.

Balance within all aspects of the human body is therefore the main aim of Chinese medicine practitioners including balance across the internal fluids, organs, and energy sources. An imbalance in just one of these can have major implications, even more so when trying to get pregnant!

Rather than focusing on a single issue, Chinese medicine is of the opinion that treating the whole body will restore balance, therefore, encouraging the body to work more efficiently. For a woman trying to get pregnant, it is imperative that a holistic view is taken, which includes looking at the spiritual, mental, and physical state, and searching for anything which could be affecting the potential for getting pregnant.

Diagnosis of the problem will allow a bespoke treatment to be formulated. This can include a wide variety of things such as altering diet, increasing movement, taking herbal supplements, or beginning acupuncture.

The Fundamental Principles of Traditional Chinese Medicine

Traditional Chinese Medicine (TCM) was established on the principles of Tao, or put simply how the world is based on the interaction of opposites. This can commonly be referred to as Yin and Yang, but why are they crucial, and what is the link between them and infertility? These two entities are opposites of energy, with one obviously being influenced by the other and it is imperative that both are in harmony if not, disease and health issues can arise.

Looking into the fundamentals of Chinese belief, everything a person eats, thinks or does affects Yin and Yang. In order to reach the perfect balance and thus optimal health, attention needs to be paid to these variables. By eating and drinking correctly and maintaining good mental health you can regulate this balance and ultimately regulate the health of your body. Most people will at some point in their life have pushed too hard at work, not slept enough, and ended up falling ill. These situations are a perfect example of how our body can end up in imbalance with one of the energies being in abundance compared to the other. Fertility is particularly delicate to the changes in the Yin and Yang energy so let's investigate this in more detail.

The uterus is benefited by Yin and therefore Yin allows the uterus to be able to successfully protect and support embryo development. Yin produces the hormone estrogen to build the walls of the womb and initiate anatomical changes such as the production of mucus which is required for the embryo to continue to develop. Everyone gets older and unfortunately, as this happens, Yin levels drop allowing the introduction of Yang (hot energy). This causes a reduction in estrogen and, during menopause, is responsible for hot flashes and sweating during sleep. If a woman wishes to achieve pregnancy when older it is imperative that the Yin energy is kept high and Yang low in order to increase the woman's fertility. This is only one of several examples of how these energies can affect fertility so let's take a deeper look.

Qi Energy: The Basis of Life

All cells allow the passing of energy throughout our body via proteins and without this there would be no supply of power to our internal organs leading to chaos. The energy which regulates this system and also the release of hormones and chemical processes is what the Chinese call "Qi".

The flow of Qi within the body is via networks known as meridians and it is these that are the focus of acupuncture specialists and allow the rerouting of any energy which may be lost within the body. Yin and Yang can be thought of as specific forms of Qi which courier energy within the body. Everything which is in your body has Qi and keeping your body balanced is dependent upon the flow of Qi and the elimination of waste products which may negatively affect this flow.

Unfortunately, in Western medicine, only one problem or related system tends to be investigated at any one time. This is contrary to TCM which considers every type of Qi to heal a problem in the body regardless of the location. An example of this would be a woman who has menstrual issues and could actually end up being treated for a liver affliction.

Addressing and curing the liver issue would in turn help the woman to conceive due to the link which exists between fertility and the liver. Chinese medicine specifically looks at the way all the organs and systems communicate as well as the need for balanced Qi.

Important Organ Systems

There are six specific organ systems that pair with associated meridians:

- The Heart
- The Lung and Large Intestines (this does not affect fertility)
- The Kidneys and Bladder
- The Spleen's Role in Digestion and Immune Function
- The Liver and Gallbladder
- The Uterus

Connection Between Heart and Uterus

When looking into the principles of Chinese medicine, the Heart is not only responsible for pumping blood around the body, it also influences the mind and spirit. This defines our personality and helps us find serenity in our way of life.

In Chinese medicine, the Heart and Uterus are connected via an internal channel called the Bao Mai (Uterus Vessel) which is responsible for the necessary blood flow to the uterus so any emotional upset which affects your Heart such as anxiety and stress, can disrupt the ability for the uterus to nourish and develop a fetus.

Kidneys and TCM

In an anatomical sense, the Kidneys are thought of as the organs which remove waste products in the body as well as regulate water balance. The Kidneys are a little more complicated in TCM however and are thought of as genetic regulators and the foundation of life. Whilst they help filter toxins from your body, they also house your willpower, govern the water and fire in your body and they're the holders of your Jing (essence). In other words, it is the Kidneys that will signal when a young girl will start having periods and will dictate what will happen all the way through to a woman beginning menopause later in life.

It is also thought in Chinese medicine that the Kidneys are directly linked to fundamental organs and systems in the body such as the nervous system, endocrine system, skeletal system, and more relevant to this book, the reproductive system.

As a result of this link, the Kidneys can also be an important tool to help cure infertility. In some cases, stimulating the Kidneys can lead to the production of follicle-stimulating hormone (FSH) which is not only important in activating the production of estrogen in the ovaries, but also allows follicles to grow. As follicles contain eggs this process is fundamental to getting pregnant. Having a diagnosis of weak Kidney energy is usually treated by acupuncture and the use of specific herbs to restore them to normal function.

The Speen's Role in Digestion and Immune Function

The official role of the Spleen, as defined by modern medicine today, is to act as a filter for the blood, produce white blood cells (lymphocytes), and help to defend the body and protect it against pathogens and other infectious agents. However, the definition given by traditional Chinese medicine is much more diverse and classifies the Spleen as a partner to the Stomach, becoming key in digestion and transporting all nutrients and energy required for the body to the four limbs.

The Spleen is also important for the organs along the midline of the body such as the uterus, bladder, and stomach as the Spleen Qi offers a lifting effect, making sure these organs are correctly situated and optimally performing. In addition, the Spleen is involved in the production of many hormones essential for conceiving and carrying to full term and for this reason, problems with the Spleen network can result in infertility.

Common causes of Spleen Qi deficiency which will stop it from working correctly are a poor diet. Eating too much or too little will damage the Spleen, for example eating too many greasy foods, carbohydrates, protein or refined sugar can cause Spleen Qi deficiency. Also, emotional strain will damage the Spleen such as stress and worrying excessively so it is important to practice relaxation techniques which will help to release trapped energy and rebalance the harmony between the thinking (Spleen) and the spirit (Heart).

Importance of the Gallbladder/Liver Function

In traditional Chinese medicine, the Liver is extremely important and is classified as the organ that has the largest impact on a woman's health. Its main role is to detoxify the blood and control the metabolism of important fertility hormones which are essential for many things, in particular ovulation.

The Liver Qi needs to flow freely and move in harmony to control and create a regular menstrual cycle. The Liver controls the flow of blood and directs it from the organs to the uterus just before menstruation begins. When the Liver Qi is stuck, this results in cramping, headaches, and negative emotions that a woman can experience during this time. In TCM Liver Qi stagnation can cause excessive menstruation and blood stagnation which can cause insufficient flow or hormonal issues. Over time, this blockage or buildup can cause changes in the endometrium of the uterus that can lead to fibroids and polyps.

The partner organ of the Liver is the Gallbladder which stores bile produced by the Liver. If either of these organs fails to work correctly, then it will significantly impact fertility as hormone levels will become imbalanced. If left untreated the Liver Qi stagnation can create an inhospitable uterine environment where eggs will fail to fertilize, fail to implant or embryos will be lost through miscarriage.

The Uterus (Palace of The Child)

A woman's uterus is known as 'Bao Gong' or 'Zi Gong' which translates to "Palace of the Child" in Chinese medicine that needs Blood and Qi to function correctly.

PreConception Miracle For Women Over 40

This very sacred region of the body is known as the lower Dan Tien where Jing and Spirit join together to create life so no wonder it is known as the elixir field or energy center of the body. The uterus has an extremely close relationship with the meridian networks and is sensitive to all disruption throughout the rest of the body. Only when all of the meridian pathways and the organs are functioning optimally can the uterus also work normally and conception occurs.

How You Can Conceive with the Help of Chinese Medicine

So by now, you understand the importance of alignment throughout the uterus and reproductive organs for conception, carrying a successful pregnancy to term, and the balance with Qi energy but what in particular can cause imbalance and should therefore be avoided?

Unfortunately, there are many things that can cause disruption of Qi and make it more difficult to achieve pregnancy. These disruptions include a bad diet, emotional states such as stress or worry, toxins and chemicals, and lack of exercise.

With such a wide range of potential disruptions it can seem like a never-ending task to identify and eliminate them all but please do not worry. Traditional Chinese medicine relies on small gentle corrections to find a balanced state and therefore over time, it is very possible to re-align any disruption.

The most difficult part of the journey is identifying what is the disturbance or in other words what organ isn't working correctly. The best way to do this is to book a session with a Chinese medicine practitioner who has the skills to identify the cause of the Qi disruption. From this point, it is easy to use Chinese medicine to help cure the symptoms and restore balance.

This is particularly true in the case of the female body and treating infertility and your chosen TCM expert will be able to design a treatment protocol that is specific to your exact issue for the best chances of success.

The Incorrect Approach of Western Medicine to Infertility

Western medicine has made infertility a multi-billion dollar business, with American couples alone spend in excess of $20 billion a year on their fertility treatments. However, looking further into the success rate of these treatments we realize that more than half of couples still fail to conceive after IVF treatment so what is the reason for this?

Western medicine uses the latest medical technology and complicated regimes of medication so you would assume it would be very simple for them to help achieve pregnancy in their patients but this simply isn't the case with failure more common than success.

Put simply, Western medicine takes a very general approach and considers only common health issues, and fails to see the intricacies that Eastern medical specialists can.

The process of IVF itself, where an egg and sperm are fertilized outside of the woman's body using medical technology can help in cases where there is a blockage present within the reproductive system however even with this process, implantation simply will not take place if the natural Qi balance is not in place throughout the body. Infertility is a much more complex issue than Western medicine would like to believe and cannot simply be fixed with medication or technology. Instead, it is important to consider the whole body and adopt a natural approach. A simple way to consider this contrast is to think of a deficiency in the body such as if your thyroid wasn't functioning correctly and you were struggling to conceive as a result.

The approach by a Western medical doctor would be to prescribe a synthetic hormone medication to help address the balance whereas a doctor of Eastern medicine would instead try to identify the fundamental issue within the body causing the thyroid to function incorrectly and instead try to restore balance and return to ideal function.

I am not trying to suggest that Western medicine should be completely avoided as there are certain technologies that are essential for health but instead, I suggest that you should consider a combined approach where Eastern and Western medicine are used together to address the imbalance within the body and tackle the root of the problem while also using the tools and technology of Western medicine where necessary.

This combined approach has been shown to be by far the best method for treating infertility.

The Infertility Questionnaire

Not only do Eastern and Western medicine have differences in their treatment approaches but they also differ when it comes to diagnosis.

The process of a Western practitioner will be to use very specific and pre-defined procedures that are often invasive while an expert in Chinese medicine will rely on their expertise to assess the full body of the patient by analyzing external symptoms and differentiating the root cause by applying 4 main methods that include: observation, smelling and listening, questioning, and tongue/pulse diagnosis.

With particular consideration to fertility, the Chinese medicine diagnosis will involve an assessment of the important organs we have discussed above; the Kidney, Spleen, Liver, and Heart as well as the Blood and the Qi, including the Yin and Yang balance. Only after this thorough diagnosis can the practitioner begin to understand the complexities of the issue and start to formulate a plan for treatment to help a patient conceive.

As well as the assessment of the body and its function the Eastern medicine assessment will usually involve the completion of an extensive questionnaire which is created to fully examine the patient's lifestyle choices and health. It is important a patient is completely honest when answering these questions and doesn't try to self-diagnose or second-guess the reasoning behind the questions.

When it comes to infertility there can be a complex network of issues and therefore when answering the questions, you may feel that your answers are overlapping or involving several different diagnostic areas but this is extremely common and isn't something you should be concerned about.

A TCM practitioner will be able to clearly interpret your answers and get an understanding of what may be causing your infertility

Kidney Yin Deficiency

Fertility issues can often be linked to Kidney Yin Deficiency, a concept rooted in Traditional Chinese Medicine (TCM). This deficiency represents an imbalance in the body, characterized by a deficiency in the cooling, moistening, and nourishing aspects of Yin energy. When Kidney Yin is deficient, it can lead to disruptions in hormonal balance, irregular menstrual cycles, and reduced reproductive function.

To improve fertility, TCM practitioners often recommend dietary and lifestyle changes, herbal remedies, and acupuncture to replenish Kidney Yin, restore overall balance, and promote optimal reproductive health.

Kidney Yang Deficiency

Fertility issues can be linked to Kidney Yang Deficiency, a concept rooted in Traditional Chinese Medicine (TCM). Kidney Yang, which represents the body's warmth and metabolic processes, is essential for maintaining normal reproductive functions. When Kidney Yang is deficient, it can lead to suboptimal hormonal balance, poor egg and sperm quality, or irregular menstrual cycles, which may contribute to difficulties in conceiving.

TCM practitioners often address this imbalance through a combination of herbal remedies, acupuncture, and lifestyle changes, aiming to restore warmth and balance in the body, thus supporting fertility and overall well-being.

Heart Qi Stagnation

Fertility issues have been linked to various factors, one of which is Heart Qi Stagnation in Traditional Chinese Medicine (TCM). Heart Qi Stagnation occurs when the flow of life force energy, or "Qi," becomes obstructed, leading to emotional and physical imbalances.

As the Heart is closely associated with emotional well-being, stagnant Heart Qi can result in anxiety, stress, and other emotional disturbances that may negatively impact fertility. By addressing Heart Qi Stagnation through holistic approaches such as acupuncture, herbal medicine, and stress management techniques, individuals may find improved overall health and enhanced fertility potential.

Blood Stagnation

Fertility issues can be impacted by Blood Stagnation (also referred to as 'Blood Stasis'), a concept rooted in Traditional Chinese Medicine (TCM). Blood Stagnation is where the blood flow is heavily restricted or there is improper circulation of blood within the body, which may lead to a variety of health concerns, including reproductive difficulties. In TCM, healthy blood flow and harmonious energy circulation are essential for optimal fertility, as they nourish the reproductive organs and support overall well-being. By addressing Blood Stagnation through acupuncture, herbal treatments, and lifestyle changes, individuals may improve their chances of conception by promoting a more balanced flow of Qi and Blood.

Phlegm/Damp Accumulation

Fertility is a complex physiological process that can be influenced by various factors, including the balance of bodily fluids in traditional Chinese medicine (TCM). Phlegm or damp accumulation, one of the fundamental TCM concepts, refers to the excessive buildup of fluids in the body, often caused by an imbalance in the body's energy or Qi.

When phlegm or dampness accumulates, it can obstruct the flow of Qi and blood, potentially impairing reproductive functions. This obstruction may lead to difficulties in conception, as the nourishment and environment necessary for healthy egg and sperm production, as well as embryo implantation, are disrupted.

To address fertility issues related to phlegm or damp accumulation, TCM practitioners often prescribe herbal remedies, acupuncture, and lifestyle changes to restore the body's balance and enhance fertility.

Spleen Qi Deficiency

Spleen Qi Deficiency is a common Traditional Chinese Medicine (TCM) diagnosis that can have a significant impact on fertility. In TCM, the Spleen is responsible for transforming and transporting vital nutrients throughout the body, as well as managing blood flow.

When Spleen Qi is deficient, the body may struggle to nourish the reproductive system properly, leading to issues such as irregular menstrual cycles, poor egg quality, and a weakened uterine lining.

By addressing and correcting Spleen Qi Deficiency through acupuncture, herbal medicine, and lifestyle changes, it is possible to restore balance and improve overall fertility.

Liver Qi Stagnation

Fertility issues can often be linked to Liver Qi Stagnation, a concept rooted in Traditional Chinese Medicine (TCM). This imbalance occurs when the flow of life energy, or Qi, within the Liver, becomes disrupted, leading to both physical and emotional symptoms. In relation to fertility, Liver Qi Stagnation can contribute to menstrual irregularities, hormonal imbalances, and even reduced egg quality. By addressing this stagnation through acupuncture, herbal remedies, or lifestyle adjustments, individuals seeking to improve their fertility may experience better overall reproductive health and an increased likelihood of conception.

Chapter 4

The 4 Menstrual Phases and the Key Processes

Introduction

Aging gracefully and achieving a healthy pregnancy after 40 can be a challenging yet fulfilling journey. Traditional Chinese Medicine (TCM) offers a holistic perspective on understanding and supporting your body through the entire menstrual cycle.

By learning about the four menstrual phases and their key processes, you can harness your body's innate wisdom to optimize your fertility.

The menstrual cycle is a vital biological process that prepares a woman's body for pregnancy every month. From a TCM perspective, the menstrual cycle reflects the delicate balance of Yin and Yang energies, Qi (vital energy), and Blood within the body.

When these energies are in harmony, fertility is enhanced, making it essential for women over 40 to maintain this equilibrium for optimal conception chances.

Hormones play a crucial role in orchestrating the menstrual cycle, and their levels fluctuate throughout each phase.

TCM emphasizes the importance of a balanced endocrine system, as hormonal imbalances can contribute to difficulties in conceiving, especially for women over 40.

1. Menstrual Phase: Shedding The Uterine Lining

As a woman in her 40s exploring fertility options, understanding your menstrual cycle is essential in optimizing your chances of conception. Traditional Chinese Medicine (TCM) offers a unique perspective on the four menstrual phases, emphasizing the importance of balance and harmony within the body to achieve optimal fertility.

Shedding the Uterine Lining: A Time of Renewal

The first phase of the menstrual cycle, shedding the uterine lining, is commonly referred to as menstruation or the period. This phase typically lasts between 3 to 7 days and is marked by the shedding of the endometrial lining that has built up during the previous cycle. In TCM, this phase is regarded as a time of renewal and cleansing, allowing the body to prepare for the possibility of pregnancy in the upcoming cycle.

The Importance of Qi and Blood

The concepts of Qi (life force or energy) and Blood are integral to understanding fertility. During the shedding phase, the focus is on ensuring a smooth flow of Qi and Blood. The proper circulation of these vital substances is essential for maintaining balance within the body and promoting optimal reproductive health. In women over 40, nurturing the Qi and Blood becomes even more critical, as age-related changes can lead to stagnation or depletion of these essential elements.

Diet and Lifestyle Recommendations

TCM emphasizes the importance of diet and lifestyle adjustments to support the shedding of the uterine lining and improve fertility. Here are some recommendations specifically tailored for women over 40:

① **Warming Foods:** Consume warming foods such as ginger, cinnamon, and soups made with bone broth to help promote the smooth flow of Qi and Blood during the shedding phase. These foods can enhance circulation and reduce stagnation, thus facilitating the proper discharge of the uterine lining.

② **Rest and Relaxation:** During menstruation, it is crucial to prioritize rest and relaxation, allowing your body the time it needs to rejuvenate. Gentle stretching or restorative yoga practices can help to calm the mind and support the flow of Qi and Blood.

③ **Avoid Cold and Raw Foods:** Cold and raw foods can constrict blood vessels, leading to stagnation and cramping during the shedding phase. Instead, focus on consuming warm, cooked foods to support the smooth flow of Qi and Blood.

④ **Hydration:** Drinking plenty of warm water, herbal teas, bone broth, and nourishing soups will help maintain optimal hydration levels and facilitate the healthy discharge of the uterine lining.

Herbal Support

Traditional Chinese Medicine utilizes a range of herbal formulas to support the menstrual cycle, particularly during the shedding phase. Some common herbs used to promote a smooth and healthy shedding of the uterine lining include:

⑤ **Dang Gui (Angelica sinensis):** Known as the "female ginseng," Dang Gui is used to nourish and invigorate the Blood, which is essential for a healthy menstrual cycle.

⑥ **Chuan Xiong (Ligusticum chuanxiong):** Chuan Xiong is a powerful herb for promoting Blood circulation and relieving pain associated with menstruation.

⑦ **Yi Mu Cao (Leonurus japonicus):** This herb is traditionally used to regulate menstruation, support the shedding of the uterine lining, and alleviate menstrual cramps.

2. Follicular Phase: Follicle Growth And Hormonal Changes

As you journey through the complexities of fertility, understanding the menstrual phases can provide valuable insights. When you reach the age of 40, conceiving may prove more challenging, but rest assured that Traditional Chinese Medicine (TCM) can support you through this delicate process.

The Follicular Phase: A Brief Overview

The follicular phase begins on the first day of your menstrual cycle, lasting until ovulation. This phase is characterized by the growth and development of ovarian follicles, which house the eggs that will be released during ovulation. Hormonal changes occur simultaneously, preparing the endometrium (uterine lining) for a potential pregnancy. The primary hormones at play during the follicular phase are follicle-stimulating hormone (FSH), luteinizing hormone (LH), and estrogen.

Traditional Chinese Medicine and the Follicular Phase

TCM sees the body as a complex, interconnected system, where the balance of Qi (energy) and blood flow is crucial for optimal health and fertility. During the follicular phase, TCM focuses on nourishing the Kidney and Liver systems, as these organs play essential roles in egg maturation and hormone regulation. By enhancing the flow of Qi and Blood to the reproductive organs, TCM aims to create an ideal environment for conception.

1. Nourishing the Kidney System

In TCM, the Kidney system is responsible for growth, development, and reproduction. As women age, Kidney Yin and Kidney Yang energies may become depleted, potentially affecting fertility. TCM practitioners use acupuncture and herbal remedies to nourish the Kidney system and support follicle growth during the follicular phase.

• **Acupuncture:** Specific acupuncture points, such as Kidney 3 (Taixi) and Kidney 7 (Fuliu), can help to balance Kidney Yin and Yang energies, promoting optimal follicle development.
• **Herbal remedies:** Herbs like Rehmannia (Shu Di Huang), Lycium (Gou Qi Zi), and Cornus (Shan Zhu Yu) can be used to nourish Kidney Yin, while herbs like Cinnamon (Rou Gui) and Eucommia (Du Zhong) can strengthen Kidney Yang.

2. Supporting the Liver System

The Liver system is responsible for maintaining a smooth flow of Qi and Blood throughout the body. When Liver Qi stagnates, it may disrupt hormonal balance and impede fertility. During the follicular phase, TCM seeks to soothe the Liver system and ensure the smooth flow of Qi and Blood to support healthy hormone levels.

• **Acupuncture:** Acupuncture points like Liver 3 (Taichong) and Liver 5 (Ligou) can help to regulate Liver Qi and promote hormonal balance.
• **Herbal remedies:** Herbs such as Bupleurum (Chai Hu), White Peony (Bai Shao), and Cyperus (Xiang Fu) can be used to soothe Liver Qi and support hormonal balance.

Dietary Recommendations for the Follicular Phase

In addition to acupuncture and herbal remedies, TCM also emphasizes the importance of a balanced diet during the follicular phase. Eating nourishing foods can support Kidney and Liver systems while providing essential nutrients for egg maturation and hormone regulation.

• **Protein:** Incorporate high-quality protein sources like lean meats, fish, eggs, and legumes to provide the necessary amino acids for hormone production and follicle development. These proteins also support Liver and Kidney function, which play a vital role in fertility.

• **Whole grains:** Whole grains such as brown rice, quinoa, and barley are rich in B vitamins, which help support hormone balance and overall reproductive health. These grains also provide fiber, which can help regulate blood sugar levels and promote a healthy body weight, both essential factors for fertility.

• **Antioxidant-rich foods:** Foods high in antioxidants, such as berries, leafy greens, and nuts, can help protect developing follicles from oxidative stress and support overall egg health. Antioxidants can also support liver function by promoting detoxification pathways.

• **Healthy fats:** Omega-3 fatty acids, found in fatty fish like salmon, walnuts, and flaxseeds, can help to reduce inflammation and promote hormonal balance. Additionally, monounsaturated fats like olive oil and avocado can support cell membrane integrity and overall reproductive health.

• **Warm and cooked foods:** In TCM, consuming warm and cooked foods can aid digestion and enhance the absorption of nutrients. This principle is especially important during the follicular phase, as your body needs vital nutrients to support follicle growth and hormone production.

Lifestyle Recommendations for the Follicular Phase

TCM also offers lifestyle advice to help support fertility during the follicular phase. By implementing these practices, you can create a more balanced and harmonious environment for conception.

• **Stress reduction:** High-stress levels can negatively impact hormone balance and overall fertility. Incorporate stress-reducing activities like yoga, meditation, and deep breathing exercises into your daily routine to help maintain a calm and centered state of mind.

• **Moderate exercise:** Engaging in moderate exercises, such as brisk walking, swimming, or tai chi, can help to support healthy blood flow and Qi circulation, both vital for reproductive health. However, avoid excessive or high-intensity workouts, as they can deplete Kidney and Liver energy and negatively impact fertility.

• **Sleep:** Prioritize sleep and aim for 7-8 hours of quality rest each night. This will support hormone regulation, as well as overall physical and emotional well-being.

• **Avoid toxins:** Limit exposure to environmental toxins, such as cigarette smoke, alcohol, and harmful chemicals, as they can negatively impact egg quality and overall fertility. Opt for organic foods and natural cleaning and personal care products when possible.

3. Ovulatory Phase: The Release Of The Mature Ovum

The Ovulatory Phase, typically occurring around day 14 of a woman's menstrual cycle, is a crucial period for women over 40 seeking to conceive. It is during this brief window of time, lasting approximately 24 to 48 hours, that the mature ovum (egg) is released from the ovary and is available for fertilization.

The focus during this phase is on promoting the smooth flow of Qi (energy) and Blood throughout the body to support the release of the mature ovum and improve the chances of conception.

The Role of Traditional Chinese Medicine in the Ovulatory Phase

By identifying imbalances in the body's Qi, Blood, and organ systems, TCM practitioners aim to restore harmony and enhance fertility potential during the Ovulatory Phase. Key TCM principles that apply during this phase include:

① **Nourishing the Kidney Yin and Yang:** In TCM, the Kidney system is closely associated with reproduction and fertility. Ensuring the balance of Kidney Yin and Yang is essential for optimal reproductive function, particularly during the Ovulatory Phase when the egg is released. Nourishing Kidney Yin supports the growth of the follicle, while Kidney Yang provides the warmth and energy required for ovulation to occur.

② **Promoting the Smooth Flow of Liver Qi:** The Liver plays a pivotal role in regulating the menstrual cycle by ensuring the smooth flow of Qi and Blood throughout the body. Emotional stress or imbalances in the Liver system can hinder the flow of Qi, leading to stagnation and potential disruptions in the Ovulatory Phase. By promoting the smooth flow of Liver Qi, TCM can help alleviate stress, improve circulation, and enhance fertility.

③ **Strengthening the Spleen and Blood:** A strong Spleen system is vital for the production and transportation of Blood and nutrients throughout the body. Proper Blood circulation and nourishment are essential for a healthy endometrial lining and successful implantation of a fertilized egg.

During the Ovulatory Phase, TCM aims to strengthen the Spleen and Blood to create a nurturing environment for conception.

TCM Techniques and Remedies for the Ovulatory Phase

① **Acupuncture:** Acupuncture can be a valuable tool in addressing fertility challenges for women over 40. By stimulating specific acupoints, TCM practitioners can help balance the body's Qi, Blood, and organ systems, improving the likelihood of a successful Ovulatory Phase. Acupuncture may also help reduce stress, which can negatively impact fertility.

② **Herbal Medicine:** TCM herbal formulas are tailored to each individual's unique constitution and imbalances. During the Ovulatory Phase, herbs may be prescribed to nourish Kidney Yin and Yang, promote the smooth flow of Liver Qi, or strengthen the Spleen and Blood, depending on the individual's specific needs.

③ **Diet and Lifestyle:** TCM emphasizes the importance of a balanced diet and healthy lifestyle in supporting fertility. Eating warming and nourishing foods, such as lean protein, whole grains, and vegetables, can help support the Ovulatory Phase. Additionally, engaging in moderate exercise and stress reduction techniques, such as meditation or tai chi, can further enhance fertility potential.

4. Luteal Phase: Progesterone Production And Preparing For Implantation

The luteal phase is considered the most important phase for women over 40 trying to conceive. It's during this phase that the body prepares for a potential pregnancy, and is heavily influenced by the production of progesterone. This hormone plays a crucial role in ensuring the right conditions for implantation and the early stages of pregnancy.

Progesterone Production and Kidney Yang

From a TCM perspective, the luteal phase is closely related to the functioning of the Kidney Yang. The Kidney Yang is responsible for warming and nourishing the body, and its energy is crucial for the production of progesterone. In women over 40, it's common for the Kidney Yang to be depleted, which can result in lower progesterone levels and a less hospitable environment for implantation.

To support the Kidney Yang and enhance progesterone production during the luteal phase, TCM practitioners often prescribe a combination of acupuncture, herbal medicine, and dietary modifications. These treatments can help to strengthen the Kidney Yang and create a more favorable environment for implantation.

Nourishing the Uterine Lining

Another key aspect of the luteal phase in TCM is nourishing the uterine lining to facilitate implantation. During this phase, the endometrium thickens and becomes rich in blood vessels, creating a nutrient-dense environment for a fertilized egg. This process is driven by the Spleen Qi, which is responsible for transforming and transporting nutrients throughout the body.

For women over 40, it's particularly important to support the Spleen Qi in order to create a healthy uterine lining. This can be achieved through a combination of acupuncture, herbs, and dietary adjustments, such as eating warming, easily digestible foods that nourish the Spleen Qi.

Stress Reduction and Liver Qi Stagnation

Stress can have a significant impact on the luteal phase and overall fertility, especially for women over 40 who may already be experiencing age-related hormonal changes. In TCM, stress is often associated with Liver Qi stagnation, which can disrupt the smooth flow of energy throughout the body, including the reproductive organs.

To address Liver Qi stagnation during the luteal phase, TCM practitioners often recommend a combination of acupuncture, herbal medicine, and stress reduction techniques, such as meditation, yoga, Qi Gong or Tai Chi. These practices can help to promote a more balanced flow of energy and create a more conducive environment for conception.

The Role of The Heart

In TCM, the Heart plays a vital role in housing the spirit and connecting with the emotions. During the luteal phase, it's important to cultivate a calm and peaceful state of mind in order to support the implantation process.

Practices such as meditation, deep breathing exercises, affirmations, and visualization techniques can help to connect with the Heart and promote emotional well-being during this phase.

The luteal phase is a critical time for women over 40 trying to conceive. By addressing Kidney Yang deficiency, supporting the Spleen Qi, reducing Liver Qi stagnation, and nurturing the Heart, Traditional Chinese Medicine offers a holistic approach to optimizing the luteal phase and enhancing fertility for women in their 40s.

To maximize the potential for success, it's important to consult with a qualified TCM practitioner who can develop a personalized treatment plan tailored to your specific needs.

Chapter 5

Optimizing Nutrition for Each Menstrual Phase: The Best Foods to Eat

Introduction

In the intricate journey of life, fertility plays a crucial role in not only bringing forth new life but also as a reflection of a woman's overall well-being. When a woman enters her 40s, the desire to conceive may become an even more significant concern as her biological clock ticks away. Alongside the challenges of age and modern lifestyle factors, the pursuit of optimal fertility has led many to seek wisdom from the ancient practices of Traditional Chinese Medicine (TCM).

In this chapter, I delve into the art and science of optimizing nutrition for each of the menstrual phases, providing insights into the best foods to eat for enhancing fertility and ensuring a harmonious balance within the body.

Traditional Chinese Medicine, a holistic healing system with a history spanning over 3,000 years, offers invaluable insights into how to maintain and enhance one's fertility, particularly for women in their 40s. At its core, TCM views the body as a complex network of energy pathways, or meridians, that need to be balanced and nourished to promote optimal health and fertility. Central to TCM is the concept of Qi, the vital life force that flows through these meridians, and the balance of Yin and Yang, which are complementary forces that govern every aspect of our physical, emotional, and spiritual well-being.

In the context of fertility, TCM emphasizes the importance of nourishing the body and maintaining a balanced internal environment to optimize conception and pregnancy. The menstrual cycle, a crucial aspect of a woman's reproductive health, can be viewed as a microcosm of her overall health and well-being which is why it is also known as the "fifth vital sign," along with blood pressure, body temperature, heart rate, and respiratory rate. We will cover the four distinct phases of the menstrual cycle - menstruation phase, follicular phase, ovulation phase, and luteal phase - and how their unique characteristics can be supported and enhanced through a careful selection of foods and dietary practices.

As women in their 40s often face the challenges of declining egg quality and hormonal imbalances, TCM-inspired nutrition can be particularly beneficial in addressing these issues. By understanding the principles of Yin and Yang, the Five Elements Theory, and the energetics of foods, women can better harness the power of their diet to support each phase of their menstrual cycle and optimize their fertility.

In this chapter, I will also provide a comprehensive guide to the best foods to eat during each menstrual phase, drawing on the rich wisdom of Traditional Chinese Medicine. I will discuss how the energetics and properties of specific foods can nourish and replenish the body, support hormonal balance, and create an optimal environment for conception. Moreover, I will offer practical tips on how to incorporate these foods into daily meals, taking into account modern lifestyle factors and personal preferences.

1. Nourishing the Menstrual Phase: Foods for Comfort and Support

In Traditional Chinese Medicine (TCM), nutrition plays a crucial role in supporting a woman's overall health and fertility, particularly for those over 40 who are trying to conceive. As previously discussed in Chapter 4, the menstrual cycle is divided into four main phases: the menstrual phase, the follicular phase, the ovulatory phase, and the luteal phase. Each phase requires specific nutrients and energy to help the body's organs function optimally and maintain balance.

This sub-chapter focuses on the menstrual phases and offers recommendations for nourishing foods that provide comfort and support for women in their 40s seeking to optimize their fertility.

Menstrual Phase: Overview

The menstrual phase, lasting approximately 3-7 days, is when a woman's body sheds the uterine lining. From a TCM perspective, the body is releasing accumulated blood and Qi, making it a crucial time to nourish and replenish these vital elements. In this phase, the body's focus is on cleansing and rejuvenation, setting the stage for a new cycle.

Key TCM Concepts in the Menstrual Phase

① **Blood:** Blood is a vital substance in TCM, responsible for nourishing and moisturizing the organs, tissues, and meridians. During the menstrual phase, it is crucial to replenish lost blood and maintain blood quality for overall health and fertility.

② **Qi:** Qi is the life force that flows through the body, providing energy for various functions. During menstruation, Qi is consumed and needs to be replenished to maintain balance and support fertility.

③ **Warming foods:** The menstrual phase is associated with the Kidney and Liver meridians, which are responsible for warming the body. Consuming warming foods helps to replenish energy and support the body's internal temperature.

④ **Yin and Yang balance:** Maintaining a balance between Yin (cooling, nourishing) and Yang (warming, activating) energies is crucial for overall health and fertility. During the menstrual phase, focus on replenishing Yin and supporting Yang energy.

Foods for Comfort and Support

① **Dark leafy greens:** Vegetables like kale, spinach, and collard greens are high in iron, which helps to replenish lost blood. These greens also contain vitamins and minerals that nourish the body and support the Liver and Kidney meridians.

② **Bone broth:** Rich in minerals and collagen, bone broth supports the health of the reproductive system, strengthens the Kidneys, and nourishes the Blood. Consuming warm bone broth can help to alleviate menstrual cramps and replenish vital nutrients.

③ **Ginger:** Ginger is a warming herb that supports the digestive system and enhances blood circulation. Incorporating ginger into meals or drinking ginger tea can help to relieve menstrual discomfort and support overall health.

④ **Red and black foods:** In TCM, red and black foods are believed to nourish the Blood and support the Kidneys. Examples include red beans, black beans, beets, blackberries, and dark cherries. Incorporate these foods into your diet during the menstrual phase to replenish lost blood and support fertility.

⑤ **Whole grains:** Whole grains like brown rice, quinoa, and barley provide B vitamins, which are essential for energy production and hormonal balance.

Consuming whole grains can help to replenish Qi and nourish the body during the menstrual phase.

⑥ **Nuts and seeds:** Nuts and seeds such as walnuts, almonds, and sesame seeds are rich in essential fatty acids, which support hormone production and balance. These foods also provide essential nutrients to nourish the body and replenish Qi.

⑦ **Fish:** Oily fish like salmon, mackerel, and sardines are high in Omega-3 fatty acids, which support hormonal balance and reduce inflammation in the body. They also provide essential nutrients that nourish the Blood and Kidneys, promoting overall reproductive health. Including fish in your diet during the menstrual phase can help replenish vital nutrients and maintain balance in the body.

⑧ **Warm soups and stews:** Comforting, warm foods like soups and stews are beneficial during the menstrual phase, as they help to replenish lost fluids and support the body's internal temperature. Ingredients such as root vegetables, mushrooms, and dark leafy greens can provide essential nutrients while also promoting relaxation and comfort.

⑨ **Berries:** Berries are rich in antioxidants, which help to combat oxidative stress and support overall health. Consuming berries during the menstrual phase can help to replenish Qi and nourish the Blood, supporting fertility and general well-being.

⑩ **Eggs:** Eggs are a great source of protein, vitamins, and minerals that nourish the body and support hormone production. They also contain choline, which is essential for liver function and overall reproductive health. Including eggs in your diet during the menstrual phase can help to replenish lost nutrients and maintain balance in the body.

Menstrual Phase Nutrients Tips

① **Stay hydrated:** Drinking plenty of water during the menstrual phase is essential to replace lost fluids and maintain overall health. Warm water or herbal teas can also help to alleviate discomfort and support the body's internal temperature.

② **Avoid cold, raw foods:** In TCM, cold and raw foods can strain the digestive system and deplete the body's energy during the menstrual phase. Instead, opt for cooked, warm foods that are easier to digest and provide nourishment.

③ **Avoid caffeine and alcohol:** Both caffeine and alcohol can disrupt hormonal balance and increase inflammation, which can negatively impact fertility. Limiting or avoiding these substances during the menstrual phase can help to maintain balance in the body and support overall health.

④ **Listen to your body:** Your body's needs may vary during the menstrual phase, so it is essential to listen to its signals and adjust your diet accordingly. If you experience cravings for specific foods, consider if they align with the TCM recommendations for this phase and whether they may provide comfort or support.

Optimizing nutrition during the menstrual phase is vital for women over 40 who are trying to conceive. By focusing on nourishing and supportive foods from a TCM perspective, women can replenish lost Blood and Qi, maintain hormonal balance, and support overall reproductive health. Incorporating these dietary recommendations and paying attention to the body's needs during the menstrual phase can provide a solid foundation for fertility and well-being.

2. Boosting the Follicular Phase: Nutrients for Follicle Development and Growth

The follicular phase is the first stage of the menstrual cycle, lasting from the first day of menstruation until ovulation. During this time, the primary focus is on nourishing and supporting the growth and maturation of the ovarian follicles, which will ultimately release the mature egg during ovulation. From the Traditional Chinese Medicine (TCM) perspective, the key to enhancing fertility for women over 40 is to optimize nutrition, focusing on foods that strengthen the body's vital energies and provide essential nutrients for follicle development.

Nourishing the Kidney Essence

In TCM, the Kidneys are considered the foundation of reproductive health and fertility, governing the growth and maturation of eggs. For women over 40, it is crucial to nourish and support the Kidney Essence to improve the quality of the ovarian follicles. Foods that are beneficial for Kidney Essence include:

• **Black sesame seeds:** Rich in essential fatty acids and minerals, black sesame seeds support kidney function and nourish follicle growth.
• **Walnuts:** Containing omega-3 fatty acids and antioxidants, walnuts are helpful in strengthening the Kidneys and improving overall reproductive health.
• **Goji berries:** These antioxidant-rich berries nourish the Kidney Essence, support the immune system, and improve the quality of the ovarian follicles.
• **Kidney beans:** High in protein, fiber, and minerals, kidney beans provide essential nutrients that strengthen the Kidneys and support follicle growth.

Supporting Liver Qi

The Liver plays a vital role in TCM by regulating the flow of Qi (vital energy) throughout the body. A smooth flow of Qi is crucial for proper hormone regulation and follicle development. Incorporate these Liver-supporting foods into your diet:

• **Leafy greens:** Spinach, kale, and other dark leafy greens are rich in vitamins, minerals, and antioxidants, which help support liver function and maintain balanced hormone levels.

• **Beets:** Beets contain betaine, a compound that supports liver detoxification, improving hormone regulation and overall reproductive health.

• **Turmeric:** This powerful anti-inflammatory spice supports liver function and helps regulate the flow of Qi in the body.

• **Lemon:** Adding lemon to water or tea can aid in liver detoxification and promote a healthy flow of Qi.

Strengthening the Spleen

In TCM, the Spleen is responsible for transforming and transporting nutrients throughout the body. A well-functioning Spleen is essential for providing the nourishment needed for follicle growth and development. Support your Spleen with these nutrient-dense foods:

• **Sweet potatoes:** Packed with vitamins, minerals, and fiber, sweet potatoes are a nourishing and easily digestible food that supports Spleen health.

• **Pumpkin:** This nutrient-rich vegetable is beneficial for Spleen function and provides essential nutrients for follicle development.

• **Barley:** As a whole grain, barley is rich in fiber and nutrients, helping to strengthen the Spleen and support overall reproductive health.

• **Ginger:** This warming spice is particularly beneficial for the Spleen, helping to stimulate digestion and the absorption of nutrients.

Balancing Blood and Essence

Adequate Blood and Essence are vital for nourishing the follicles and promoting healthy egg development. Focus on incorporating Blood-building foods into your diet to support fertility:

• **Red meat:** Lean cuts of beef and lamb provide iron, protein, and other essential nutrients that support blood production and overall reproductive health.
• **Leafy greens:** As mentioned earlier, dark leafy greens like spinach and kale are rich in iron and other vital nutrients that help build and maintain healthy blood.
• **Blackstrap molasses:** A natural source of iron, blackstrap molasses can be added to tea or used as a sweetener in recipes to support blood production and overall reproductive health.

Emphasizing High-quality Protein

High-quality protein is essential for the growth and development of healthy follicles. As you age, your body's ability to synthesize protein declines, making it even more important to include adequate protein sources in your diet. Consider incorporating these protein-rich foods:

• **Organic chicken:** A lean source of protein, organic chicken is easily digestible and provides essential nutrients needed for follicle growth.
• **Fish:** Rich in omega-3 fatty acids and high-quality protein, fish like salmon, sardines, and mackerel support hormone balance and reproductive health.
• **Legumes:** Beans, lentils, and chickpeas are excellent plant-based sources of protein and provide essential nutrients that promote follicle development.

Including Healthy Fats

Healthy fats play a vital role in hormone production and regulation, which is essential for follicle development and overall fertility. Focus on incorporating these sources of healthy fats into your diet:

• **Avocado:** Rich in monounsaturated fats and essential nutrients, avocados support hormone balance and reproductive health.

• **Olive oil:** Using extra virgin olive oil in your cooking provides healthy fats that promote hormone balance and support overall fertility.

• **Nuts and seeds:** Almonds, chia seeds, and flaxseeds are rich in healthy fats and essential nutrients, which support hormone regulation and follicle growth.

Encouraging Warmth and Circulation

In TCM, proper circulation of Blood and energy is essential for supporting fertility. Warm foods and spices can help promote circulation and support follicle development:

• **Cinnamon:** This warming spice helps stimulate blood flow, encouraging the delivery of nutrients to the ovarian follicles.

• **Ginger:** As mentioned earlier, ginger promotes digestion and absorption of nutrients while also improving circulation.

• **Bone broth:** Rich in nutrients and collagen, bone broth supports circulation, strengthens the reproductive system, and provides essential nutrients for follicle development.

Optimizing nutrition during the follicular phase is essential for women over 40 who are trying to conceive. By focusing on nutrient-dense foods that support the Kidneys, Liver, Spleen, and Blood, you can create an optimal environment for follicle growth and development.

Emphasizing a balanced diet that incorporates high-quality protein, healthy fats, and warming foods can help improve fertility and support overall reproductive health from a Traditional Chinese Medicine perspective.

3. Fueling the Ovulatory Phase: Foods to Enhance Hormone Balance and Ovulation

The ovulatory phase is a critical period in a woman's menstrual cycle, particularly when trying to conceive. This phase is characterized by the release of a mature egg from the ovary, which then travels down the fallopian tube, where it may be fertilized by sperm. A well-balanced hormone level is essential during this time, as it influences the regularity and quality of ovulation.

Traditional Chinese Medicine (TCM) has long emphasized the importance of proper nutrition for enhancing fertility, particularly in women over 40. In TCM, the concept of Yin and Yang is used to explain the delicate balance that must be maintained in the body for optimal health and fertility. During the ovulatory phase, it is crucial to focus on nourishing Yin energy and supporting hormone balance.

Leafy Green Vegetables

Leafy green vegetables, such as spinach, kale, and bok choy, are packed with essential vitamins and minerals that can help support hormone balance and overall reproductive health. These vegetables are rich in iron, calcium, and magnesium, which play crucial roles in the regulation of hormones and the menstrual cycle.

They also contain folate, a vital nutrient for women trying to conceive, as it helps prevent neural tube defects in the developing fetus. In TCM, leafy greens are considered to be cooling and Yin-nourishing, making them an excellent food choice during the ovulatory phase.

Seeds and Nuts

Seeds and nuts, such as flaxseeds, chia seeds, pumpkin seeds, walnuts, and almonds, are rich in omega-3 fatty acids, which are essential for hormone production and overall reproductive health. They also contain essential minerals, such as zinc and selenium, which are important for supporting fertility in women over 40. In TCM, seeds and nuts are considered to be tonics for the Kidney and Liver systems, which are responsible for regulating hormone balance and maintaining reproductive health.

Fish and Seafood

Fish and seafood are rich sources of omega-3 fatty acids, which have been linked to improved hormonal balance and fertility. Fish like salmon, mackerel, and sardines are particularly beneficial during the ovulatory phase, as they contain high levels of EPA and DHA, two omega-3 fatty acids that are crucial for hormone production and healthy cell development. In TCM, fish and seafood are believed to strengthen Kidney Yin energy, promoting optimal hormone balance and reproductive health.

Berries and Antioxidant-Rich Fruits

Berries, such as blueberries, blackberries, strawberries, and raspberries, and other antioxidant-rich fruits, like pomegranates and cherries, help support hormonal balance by neutralizing free radicals and reducing oxidative stress in the body. This is particularly important for women over 40, as oxidative stress can contribute to age-related fertility decline. In TCM, these fruits are considered to be cooling and Yin-nourishing, making them an ideal choice during the ovulatory phase.

Whole Grains

Whole grains, such as brown rice, quinoa, and oats, provide essential nutrients like B vitamins, which are vital for hormone production and regulation. They also contain fiber, which can help stabilize blood sugar levels and promote healthy hormone balance. In TCM, whole grains are considered to be nourishing to the Spleen and Stomach systems, which are responsible for transforming and transporting nutrients throughout the body. A well-nourished Spleen and Stomach system can support the proper functioning of the Kidney and Liver systems, which in turn regulate hormone balance and maintain reproductive health. Including whole grains in your diet during the ovulatory phase can help provide the necessary energy and nutrients for optimal hormone balance.

Beans and Legumes

Beans and legumes, such as lentils, chickpeas, and black beans, are excellent sources of plant-based protein and essential nutrients for hormone regulation. They contain vitamins and minerals like iron, zinc, and magnesium, which can help support fertility in women over 40. In TCM, beans and legumes are considered to be nourishing for the Kidney system, which is closely linked to reproductive health and hormone balance.

Lean Protein

Incorporating lean protein sources, such as grass-fed beef, organic chicken, turkey, or tofu, into your diet during the ovulatory phase can help maintain stable hormone levels and support overall reproductive health. Protein is essential for the production and regulation of hormones, as well as the development of healthy eggs and embryos. In TCM, lean protein sources are believed to strengthen the Spleen and Stomach systems, which are necessary for proper hormone regulation and reproductive function.

Hydration

Staying well-hydrated is crucial for overall health and well-being, and it plays a significant role in maintaining hormonal balance. Drinking plenty of water and other hydrating beverages, such as herbal teas and fresh juices, can help flush toxins from the body and promote optimal kidney function.

In TCM, water is considered the most essential element for nourishing Yin energy and supporting the Kidney system, which is responsible for regulating hormone balance and reproductive health.

Incorporating these nourishing foods into your diet during the ovulatory phase can help support hormone balance and optimize fertility, particularly for women over 40. Traditional Chinese Medicine emphasizes the importance of a balanced diet in maintaining overall health and well-being, and the specific dietary recommendations discussed in this sub-chapter are designed to promote optimal hormone balance and reproductive health during the ovulatory phase.

4. Supporting the Luteal Phase: Nutritional Choices for Progesterone Production and Implantation

During this phase, which typically lasts from 12 to 16 days, progesterone production increases, and the uterine lining thickens to prepare for potential embryo implantation. As a woman in her 40s, understanding how to optimize your nutrition during this phase can significantly impact your fertility journey. In this subchapter, I will discuss the best foods and dietary practices to support progesterone production and implantation from a TCM perspective.

Warming Foods

In TCM, the luteal phase is associated with the Yang energy, which is warm and active. To support the Yang energy and encourage a healthy luteal phase, consume warming foods that are believed to boost progesterone production and promote a receptive uterine environment. Some examples of warming foods include:

• Root vegetables such as sweet potatoes, carrots, and beets
• High-quality proteins like organic chicken, turkey, or lamb
• Warming spices like cinnamon, ginger, and cloves
• Seeds, especially sunflower seeds and sesame seeds

Blood-Nourishing Foods

Adequate blood supply is essential for a healthy uterine lining and successful implantation. Blood-nourishing foods are believed to support the endometrial lining, providing the necessary nutrients for embryo implantation. Include the following blood-nourishing foods in your diet:

• Leafy green vegetables like spinach, kale, silverbeet, and Swiss chard
• Iron-rich foods like red meat, liver, and oysters
• Blackstrap molasses, a natural sweetener rich in iron and other minerals
• Foods high in vitamin C, such as kiwi, oranges, and bell peppers, which help with iron absorption

Kidney-Supportive Foods

In TCM, the kidneys are believed to play a vital role in reproductive health, particularly for women over 40. Supporting kidney function can aid in maintaining a healthy hormonal balance, including progesterone levels. Include Kidney-supportive foods in your diet, such as:

- Black beans and kidney beans
- Fish, particularly salmon, sardines, and mackerel
- Seaweed and sea vegetables
- Walnuts and black sesame seeds

Foods Rich in Healthy Fats

Healthy fats are essential for hormone production, including progesterone. Consuming foods rich in healthy fats during the luteal phase can promote hormonal balance and support fertility. Examples of healthy fats include:

- Avocado
- Coconut oil and olive oil
- Nuts, particularly almonds, walnuts, and cashews
- Fatty fish like salmon, mackerel, and sardines
- Avoid cold and raw Foods

During the luteal phase, it is essential to avoid cold and raw foods, which can cause the body's energy to become stagnant, negatively impacting the Yang energy. Some examples of cold and raw foods to avoid include:

- Raw vegetables and fruits
- Cold drinks, smoothies, ice cream, and gelato
- Sushi and other raw fish dishes

As a woman in your 40s trying to conceive, optimizing your nutrition during each of the menstrual phases is crucial.

By focusing on warming, Blood-nourishing, Kidney-supportive, and hormone-balancing foods during the luteal phase, you can support progesterone production and create a receptive environment for implantation.

Chapter 6

Conceiving Guidelines for Women Over 40

Nutrition Guidelines

To optimize the chances of conception and create a nourishing environment for a baby, it is essential to follow dietary guidelines. These guidelines are based on common dietary wisdom from both mainstream and TCM principles, supported by research, to help you conceive a healthy baby. In summary, these guidelines recommend eliminating foods that negatively impact the body, such as alcohol, caffeine, and processed sugar.

Always remember these guidelines:
• Include foods that benefit, nourish, and heal, such as vegetables, beans, and whole grains in your diet.

• Opt for warm foods to avoid overtaxing your digestion, and avoid overly spicy foods and cold beverages. Salads can be an exception.

• Avoid hard-to-digest foods, including dairy products.

• Stay away from raw meat and fish as they can harbor bacteria.

• Eat as much unprocessed, seasonal organic food as you can.

• Fill your plate with colorful fruits and vegetables. We want a rainbow of color.

• Don't be afraid of carbohydrates! We need them to ovulate and to balance hormones.

• Add more leafy green vegetables as they contain folate (vitamin B9) which is important for preventing birth defects and is a vital ingredient for healthy sperm and eggs.

• Yes to more cruciferous vegetables such as broccoli, cabbage, cauliflower, Brussel sprouts and bok choy as they contain a phytonutrient called DIM which helps with estrogen metabolism and prevents fibroids and endometriosis.

• Include healthy sources of fat in your diet such as olive oil, nuts, seeds, avocado and fatty fish. They assist in forming cell membranes and the production of hormones.

• Get the right amount of protein such as meat, fish, eggs, lentils, beans, and quinoa because the amino acids in protein is vital for egg and sperm production, and they are essential to support the normal growth of a developing embryo and the placenta.

Overall, following these dietary guidelines will contribute to a general healthy balance and optimize your fertility. Remember when you are healthy, fertility is your natural state!

Suggestions for Adhering to the Dietary Guidelines

By following these guidelines, you can avoid most refined carbohydrates, keep your blood sugar stable, and maximize nutritional value. Eating is both a habit and an essential function, which can make it difficult to change.

The guidelines are backed by research, but it's essential to follow only what makes sense for you.

Eliminating one to three items at a time over a few weeks is a more comfortable way to ease into the Dietary Guidelines than going cold turkey, which can be daunting.

Be patient and give your body time to adjust. It typically takes two to three weeks for old cravings to subside and the body to cleanse. Stick to the diet closely during this time and afterward, as well. It usually takes about three months for your body to respond fully to the changes.

Diet alone is not enough; prioritize rest and stress reduction.

Avoid using the Dietary Guidelines solely for weight loss; focus on nourishing and healing your body.

Don't let yourself go hungry, as this can stress the body.

The Dietary Guidelines should leave you feeling satisfied and fulfilled.

If you're concerned about your weight, refer to the section on maintaining a healthy BMI.

Alcohol's Impact on Fertility

Although a glass of wine can be a nice way to unwind and de-stress at the end of the day or during social gatherings, it's not a body-friendly way to cope if you're trying to conceive. In fact, alcohol needs to be eliminated entirely.

To your body, alcohol is a toxin that can disrupt nutrient absorption, weaken your immune system, and create more work for your liver. Alcohol also raises prolactin levels, which can interfere with ovulation. Prolactin is the hormone that stimulates breast milk and inhibits ovulation.

Studies have shown that even one alcoholic drink per week can significantly reduce a couple's chances of conceiving. Therefore, men should avoid alcohol or at least moderate their consumption. Excessive alcohol use can result in a rise in estrogen levels, which can interfere with sperm development and hormone levels.

Even moderate drinking (one to two drinks per day) can reduce testosterone levels and sperm counts, as well as raise the number of abnormal sperm. Moreover, alcohol is a toxin that can kill off the sperm-generating cells in the testicles. Therefore, it's better to cut it out entirely than to take any chances when trying to conceive.

Avoid Caffeine

It's crucial to remove caffeine from your diet completely, including coffee, tea, chocolate, and soda (unfortunately). Caffeine not only has a negative impact onfertility, but it also increases the risk of miscarriage, raises blood pressure, and disrupts the stress-free state required for conception. Even decaffeinated versions of coffee and tea contain some amount of caffeine, and harsh chemicals are usually used in the decaffeination process of coffee. Therefore, it's best to eliminate all coffee from your diet.

I understand how difficult it can be for those who are addicted to caffeine, as I was once in the same position. However, it's essential to take this step for your well-being. If it takes two to four weeks to wean off caffeine, that's okay. You'll experience better sleep, improved health, and increased energy without caffeine.

Avoiding Refined Sweeteners

Apart from alcohol, sugar is one of the most crucial ingredients to eliminate when trying to conceive. For those with a sweet tooth, it can be the most challenging to give up. Sugar negatively affects blood sugar and insulin levels, leading to hormonal imbalances, and can also weaken the immune system - not good news.

Unfortunately, sugar has become an added ingredient in almost everything, including bread, cereals, and many off-the-shelf products. On reading the label, you might see "cane sugar," "brown sugar," "high fructose corn syrup," or just plain "sugar" listed as one of the ingredients. It's best not to buy these products and instead stick to whole grains, fruits, and vegetables - some of which have natural sugars in them.

Health food stores often carry wholesome products that don't contain processed sugar, including sugar-free, wheat-free, and yeast-free bread.

If eliminating sugar from your diet proves challenging, try using stevia. Stevia is a natural herb that's said to be 10 to 15 times sweeter than table sugar and has a negligible effect on blood sugar levels. You can find stevia in powder or liquid form at your local health food store, but be sure to check the labels for added maltodextrin and silica. Opt for pure stevia extract whenever possible.

Natural Sugars in Balanced Amounts are Beneficial

Moderate consumption (up to three tablespoons in a day) of natural sugars such as honey, maple syrup, and brown rice syrup doesn't adversely affect blood sugar levels.

However, it's best to choose organic and all-natural varieties with no added ingredients (be sure to check labels).

It's difficult to determine how much of these natural sweeteners are added to packaged foods, so it's best to eliminate such foods or consume them only in small amounts, occasionally. Whole fruits are a good source of nutrients and are beneficial for your health. However, fruit juices should be avoided or consumed only in small amounts after being diluted with water. The concentration of sugar in fruit juices is too high.

Jam should also be avoided for the same reason, even if it's all-natural and contains only fruit and fruit juice concentrate.

Avoid Artificial Sweeteners

It's best to avoid artificial sweeteners as they're not natural and can harm your reproductive health. Opt for natural sweeteners instead.

Avoid Dairy

Eliminate milk, cheese, and other dairy products as they have been linked to a decrease in fertility. Dairy can negatively affect your endocrine and immune systems, producing galactose, which is harmful to human eggs. Additionally, lactose intolerance is common, and most adults can no longer digest it. This makes it harder for your body to digest dairy products. If you notice a positive change in your health after giving up dairy, consider eliminating it for good.

If you need a milk substitute, try almond, oat, coconut, macadamia or rice milk, but be cautious about soy intake. If you must have dairy occasionally, choose organic products to avoid hormones and other additives. Calcium-rich alternatives include leafy greens like broccoli, kale, and spinach, oranges, black beans, salmon, sesame seeds, and almonds.

Yogurt is the only dairy product you may consider keeping in your diet. Organic, minimally processed yogurt with live cultures can aid in combating candida and yeast infections. Always check the label for added ingredients, especially sugar.

Avoid Wheat

Beyond the sensitivity concern, wheat can be difficult for our bodies to digest, something we want to avoid when trying to conceive. It can also have an acidic effect on the body, which is undesirable since we strive to maintain a more alkaline pH balance for good health and fertility.

Consequently, it is essential to eliminate wheat from our diet. However, this may mean giving up our favorite bread, baked goods, crackers, tortillas, pasta, and more. Moreover, wheat can be a "hidden" ingredient in several processed foods, such as soy sauce.

Fortunately, many non-wheat alternatives are now available at local health food stores and online. These include gluten-free breads, rice pasta, spelt tortillas, and non-wheat soy sauce (Tamari). Other grains like quinoa, rice, and spelt can also be substituted for wheat. Spelt, for example, is similar to wheat, but contains more protein and is easier to digest.

To determine whether a food item contains wheat, examine the list of ingredients provided on the label. Wheat may appear in various forms, such as flour, white flour, whole wheat flour, semolina, durum, triticale (a blend of wheat and rye), bran (or wheat bran), bulgur (or bulghur wheat), garam (wheat flour), wheat germ, and wheat starch. Certain dishes like couscous and tabbouleh are also made from wheat-based ingredients.

However, there is one exception I make for wheatgrass juice, which is loaded with numerous health benefits, including one that helps with fertility.

Rejecting the Majority of Highly Processed Food Items

Processed foods are those that have been modified from their natural state, typically for convenience or safety purposes. Unfortunately, most processed foods contain preservatives, artificial ingredients, and unhealthy saturated or trans fats. Additionally, much of the nutrients have been stripped away during processing, which can lead to various health problems and strain on your liver and digestive system.

What can you do? Avoid packaged, canned, or bottled foods as much as possible. This means steering clear of prepared meals, canned meats, and even deli meats, which often contain preservatives such as nitrates or nitrites.

However, some minimally processed foods are acceptable. For instance, rice noodles with just rice and water are perfectly fine. Gluten-free pasta like rice pasta, quinoa pasta, soba noodles, or chickpea pasta is also a good option. A package of oatmeal containing only whole-grain oats with no additives is another example of a healthy choice. Frozen vegetables are a decent alternative when fresh ones aren't available or when pressed for time, but ensure that the package contains only the vegetables without any additives.

When grocery shopping, read the list of ingredients on every package and ensure that there are only a few simple ingredients, all of which are permitted on this diet.

If an ingredient is unfamiliar, write it down and research it online to learn more. Avoid foods that contain partially hydrogenated vegetable oil or vegetable shortening, which translates to trans fats and is particularly harmful to your health. Also, steer clear of foods that contain preservatives, artificial colors or flavors, added sugar, or anything beyond basic whole ingredients.

Choose Pure Filtered Water Only

Drinking ample amounts of clean, filtered water is crucial to maintaining a healthy body. As water constitutes 70 percent of our body composition and has an alkalizing effect on our systems, it is recommended to consume at least six to eight 8-ounce glasses of water every day. It is vital to emphasize the word "filtered" as even bottled spring water may contain impurities like pentachlorophenol (PCP), a contaminant found in herbicides, insecticides, and industrial waste sites.

This fact is quite alarming. In July 2009, when the Subcommittee on Oversight and Investigations scrutinized the quality of bottled water, its chairman, Bart Stupak (Democratic congressman, Michigan), revealed that bottled water had been recalled because of contamination caused by arsenic, bromate, cleaning compounds, mold, and bacteria.

If you are preparing your body for a baby, you must avoid such pollutants at all costs. Instead, go for bottled water that has gone through a process of "reverse osmosis" or "distillation" to purify it (it should say this on the packaging), or be sure to use a good filter over your tap water.

The Food and Drug Administration (FDA) has concluded that the plastic utilized in disposable water bottles presents no significant threat to human health, as only trivial quantities of potentially hazardous chemicals leach from the plastic into the water. Nevertheless, a 2009 study conducted in Germany has cast doubts on this safety assessment. The research provides proof that estrogenic compounds (endocrine disruptors) seep from the plastic into the water, which can be detrimental to reproductive hormones. The study's authors assert that additional research is necessary to establish the level of health risk this may pose to humans. Until more information is available, it may be prudent to use alternative types of containers, such as glass, steel, or aluminum, for carrying water.

Resist the Temptation of Non-Essential Drinks

The majority of the beverages available in the market today are loaded with artificial ingredients, preservatives, additives, and/or added sugar. It's best to avoid them, especially sodas, even if they claim to be sugar-free and caffeine-free. Your body does not require these artificial components. Apart from purified water, herbal tea is a good alternative that is naturally caffeine-free.

However, avoid herbal teas that are not recommended during pregnancy or for fertility, such as chamomile, Echinacea, St John's wort, ginkgo biloba (the latter three also for men). Raspberry Leaf tea is believed to aid fertility by toning the uterus but it's also believed to induce contractions. Hence, it's advisable to consume it during pre-ovulation and readiness for conception, but not post-ovulation.

Fresh vegetable juice is wholesome and nutritious, especially when made at home or at a juice stand and consumed immediately. The packaged variety, even if flash pasteurized, won't have the same nutritional value. Check labels to ensure that there are no additives, and remember that cold juice will require extra energy from your body for digestion. Heating up your juice or letting it come to room temperature can reduce this extra work.

It's best to avoid iced and cold drinks and opt for beverages closer to body temperature. You can even warm up your water to aid digestion. Fruit juice should also be avoided due to its high sugar content. Instead, consume whole fruits.

Lastly, consuming one ounce of wheatgrass juice daily is said to clean the blood, aid in cell regeneration, and be a good source of chlorophyll and folate. The high magnesium content in its chlorophyll is also believed to build enzymes that restore sex hormones.

Organic Food for Fertility

It's important to prioritize eating organic whenever possible. The USDA requires organic foods to be produced without the use of harmful pesticides, synthetic fertilizers, sewage sludge, bioengineering, or ionizing radiation, all of which can have negative impacts on your health and fertility. Despite being more expensive and harder to find, your body deserves and needs the benefits of organic food.

When it comes to produce and meat, organic is a must. Non-organic produce often contains high levels of pesticides and other chemicals, while conventionally raised meat can contain growth hormones, antibiotics, additives, and preservatives that negatively affect our hormones.

Additionally, ranchers may feed cows non-organic feed that includes other meat or beef parts, which has been implicated in causing mad cow disease. It's crucial to avoid these harmful substances while nurturing your body for pregnancy.

Organic Vegetables and Fruits

When it comes to food, vegetables are a category that you should indulge in without restraint. Have as much as you like, but make sure you consume 7 plus servings of vegetables and 2-3 servings of fruit daily. Vegetables are rich in vital nutrients such as fiber, vitamins, and minerals, and help regulate blood sugar levels, which is crucial for   fertility. Eating a variety of vegetables of different colors offers a broad range of nutritional benefits.

Leafy greens like kale, spinach, chard, and celery are rich in folate, which is essential for fertility and preventing certain birth defects. In addition, these vegetables contain vitamins A, B, C, calcium, beta-carotene, iron, and many other nutrients.

Steaming vegetables is a great way to release nutrients and make them easier to digest, but overcooking them can lead to a loss of nutrients. Salads are an excellent way to consume vegetables, but don't overdo it as your body needs to expend extra energy to digest them.

Potatoes, on the other hand, are starchy and have a "fast" effect on blood sugar, so it's best to eat them boiled or steamed and combine them with other sources of healthy fiber.

Fruits are also essential sources of vitamins, bioflavonoids, and antioxidants that help counteract the effects of free radicals, which damage cells. As with vegetables, try to eat as much variety and as many colors of fruits as possible, but limit consumption to about four servings per day.

Fruit juices should be avoided as they contain high sugar concentrations. Avocados are considered the fertility fruit because they are packed with folate, "good" heart-healthy fats, and enzymes that aid digestion.

It's best to eat only organic fruits and vegetables. Conventional versions may contain chemicals and pesticides that can be harmful to your body.

Choose Organic Whole Grains

Organic whole grains are comprised of three parts: the bran, endosperm, and germ. They contain antioxidants, iron, and B vitamins and include buckwheat, wild rice, oatmeal, brown rice, whole grain barley, Kamut, and others. They are also used in food items such as cereal, crackers, and flour.

Compared to refined grains that have had their outer layer removed (although manufacturers sometimes add back lost nutrients), whole grains contain more essential nutrients and fiber, which can help stabilize blood sugar levels, beneficial for fertility.

For maximum nutritional benefits, try incorporating as many non-wheat whole grains as possible. However, they may be more challenging to digest compared to refined grains such as white rice, as they require more time and effort for your digestive system to break down. Whole grains that have been crushed into flour are easier to digest but may have lost some of their blood sugar stabilizing effect.

Overall, it's essential to consider the nutritional and blood sugar effects of the food you consume. If you're following a diet that excludes wheat, sugar, and highly processed foods while consuming plenty of vegetables, fruits, and beans, these choices are already supporting your blood sugar and nutrient needs.

White basmati rice, which has a moderate impact on blood sugar, is the preferred rice choice for recipes, but you can occasionally mix it up with brown rice (a whole grain) or even better, alternative grains such as quinoa or spelt.

Whole grains are more nutritious, but refined grains such as white rice are easier to digest. Avoid consuming large amounts of white rice on an empty stomach without other foods. It's all about balance!

Healthy Fats and Oils

Fat is crucial for our bodies, especially when we're trying to conceive. It plays a vital role in our endocrine function, which regulates the hormones necessary for reproduction. Additionally, fat is where estrogen is produced and stored. So, this is not the time to be on a low-fat diet! Fats also have a satiating effect that can help curb hunger.

However, it's essential to know which fats to consume since some are good while others are not. The worst type of fat that you should eliminate from your diet for life is trans fat. These fats, also labeled as "hydrogenated oil" or "partially hydrogenated oil" on packaging, are not natural, and our body does not require them.

Manufactured to stabilize liquid oils and prolong shelf life, trans fats are present in an overwhelming number of packaged foods, even those labeled as "natural" or "healthy." They are also present in margarine and deep-fried foods at restaurants. Trans fats pose significant health concerns, so it's crucial to check labels and eliminate them.

Saturated fats, mostly found in meat and dairy products (and in small amounts in vegetable oils), increase harmful LDL cholesterol and should be avoided. If you consume meat, opt for lean cuts. When purchasing processed products like sauces and salad dressings, check the labels for saturated fat content, additives, and preservatives, and avoid or eliminate these.

Interestingly, our bodies can produce saturated fat if we consume enough healthy fats, so we don't need to consume it. The "good" fats are monounsaturated and polyunsaturated fats, which have numerous health benefits when consumed in moderation. They reduce blood pressure, stabilize blood sugar levels, ease inflammation, and as a result, boost fertility. Avocados, nuts, and olive oil are excellent sources of healthy monounsaturated fats.

Omega-3 fatty acids are polyunsaturated fats that provide essential nutrients and have numerous health benefits.

Since our bodies cannot produce them, we must obtain them from food. Excellent sources include flaxseeds, walnuts, and seafood. Plain olive oil is the best option for all types of cooking, and it has the most antioxidants and nutrients and the best, richest flavor.

For cold dishes like salads, flaxseed oil (which should never be heated), extra virgin olive oil, and nut oils like walnut or almond are healthy choices. Among the olive oils, extra virgin is the healthiest, and it's safe to use for stir-frying or sautéing but should never be used for high-temperature cooking like deep-frying or baking. It breaks down at high temperatures, so I only recommend using it cold, on salads, or fresh tomatoes with basil, for example.

It's essential to note that even good fats can become bad if they're damaged by excessive heat, light, or oxygen. Polyunsaturated fats tend to be the most fragile, so oils that are high in polyunsaturated fats, like flaxseed, safflower, and sunflower, should be refrigerated. Their packaging should indicate this. All oils should be stored in a dark, cool place. When choosing fats and oils, it's best to opt for organic choices.

Organic Lean Meat for Fertility

To optimize fertility, it is important to consume meat and poultry as they are rich sources of protein, selenium, and essential B vitamins. However, it is crucial to opt for organic, lean varieties. Organic meat is free from growth hormones and antibiotics that can negatively impact our hormones and fertility.

Ranchers who label their meat organic must ensure their livestock are fed an organic, vegetarian diet free of chemicals, additives, and genetically modified foods, which is easier on our digestive and immune systems.

When it comes to meat, it is important to choose lean cuts as long-term pesticide residues and toxic byproducts of manufacturing such as dioxins tend to settle in the fat of the animal. In the case of poultry, it is advisable to remove the skin which can retain chemicals. If organic meat is difficult to locate, it is recommended to look for all-natural meat that is free from antibiotics, growth hormones, preservatives, and additives. If the animals have been fed an all-vegetable diet, it is preferable. Although the feed may not be organic, it is not as important.

When purchasing meat, it is important to inquire about antibiotics, growth hormones, and organic certification. For those having trouble finding organic meat, there are options available online or at stores like Whole Foods Market.

It is advised to limit red meat intake to one or two servings per week as it is high in saturated fat and harder to digest. For poultry, it is recommended to choose light meat like the breast which is lower in fat and easier to digest. For pork, fresh lean cuts like tenderloin, loin chops, and sirloin roast are preferable while avoiding fatty or processed versions of pork like bacon.

Processed meat like hot dogs, canned chicken, and most sandwich meat should be avoided altogether as they contain preservatives, additives, nitrates, nitrites, and other inferior meat products which can be harmful. Additionally, raw or undercooked meat should not be consumed as it can harbor harmful bacteria. Remember, what you put in your body has an impact on your fertility and the health of your baby.

Seafood

Seafood is a great source of healthy fats, lean protein, B vitamins, and essential minerals like iron, zinc, iodine, and selenium. However, it's important to limit your intake to once or twice per week due to mercury levels. It's a shame to restrict your intake because of the benefits, but choosing seafood with lower mercury levels can help. Opt for halibut and wild-caught salmon as they contain the lowest levels of mercury. Zinc, found in oysters, is also an important mineral for both male and female fertility.

Nuts and Seeds

Nuts and seeds are nutrient-dense and are an important part of fertility nutrition, pregnancy nutrition, and beyond, because they supply the body with ample fiber, protein, selenium, zinc, magnesium, vitamin E, and essential fatty acids. For optimal fertility benefits, pumpkin and sesame seeds are excellent choices as they contain high levels of monounsaturated fats and zinc, a crucial nutrient for male and female reproduction. Flaxseeds are also beneficial due to their abundance of omega-3 fats, which are essential for the body but cannot be produced independently. Flaxseed oil is an excellent addition to salads, but it should never be heated. Furthermore, flaxseeds are an excellent source of folate.

Almonds and walnuts are the best nuts for fertility, as almonds provide healthy monounsaturated fats while walnuts are an excellent source of omega-3 fats and essential nutrients. Brazil nuts are one of the best sources of selenium, which is good for both sperm and eggs as well as the endometrial lining.

You can sprinkle nuts and seeds on salads or add them to oatmeal. Eating nuts and seeds raw and whole may require more effort to digest; however, there are numerous health benefits for fertility. Soaking almonds in water before eating makes them easier to digest, and crushing nuts before adding them to food can also aid digestion.

To ensure freshness, buy and eat organic, raw nuts and seeds, and store them in the refrigerator. Since they are high in fat, it's best to consume no more than two ounces (about a ½ cup in volume) a day.

Beans Boost Fertility

Beans and legumes are an excellent choice for promoting fertility due to their high nutrient content. They are rich in protein, fiber, calcium, iron, potassium, and folate. Folate, in particular, is beneficial for fertility in both men and women, and it can also prevent certain birth defects.

In addition, beans are low in fat and are good for digestion and heart health. Their high fiber content helps to stabilize blood sugar levels, and they also contain antioxidants.

The level of antioxidant activity varies with the seed coat color, with black beans having the highest, followed by red, brown, yellow, and white beans. However, green peas and snow peas should be avoided as they contain a natural contraceptive called m-xylohydroquinine, which interferes with estrogen and progesterone. This contraceptive is not present in other legumes, so feel free to enjoy them.

Limit Soy

Soybeans are a great source of protein, as they contain a complete set of amino acids. They are also rich in magnesium, iron, omega-3 fatty acids, and other nutrients, making them a popular food for their many health benefits. However, when you give up dairy, you may be tempted to consume a lot of soy products, such as soy milk, soy cheese, tofu, tempeh, soy burgers, and soy chips.

This is not advisable, as many of these are processed foods. Soybeans contain isoflavones, which can mimic estrogen in large or concentrated amounts and negatively affect fertility.

Additionally, processed soy has been linked to impaired mineral absorption and thyroid dysfunction, both of which are detrimental to conception.

It is recommended that you limit your soy consumption to no more than three servings per week and choose whole soy foods, such as tofu, soy milk, and edamame, for optimal nutrition. Fermented soy products, like tofu, miso, and soy sauce, are also a better choice than processed soy, according to research.

How to Optimize Water for Digestion

To aid digestion, it's best to avoid consuming large quantities of water or any beverage during your meal as the hydrochloric acid in your stomach is working to break down your food. It disrupts the digestion process. It's recommended to drink water one hour prior to your meal and wait at least an hour after your meal to drink again. However, taking small sips during your meal is acceptable.

Achieving Optimal pH Levels

Maintaining a slightly alkaline environment is crucial for optimal health in our bodies. However, certain foods like meat and nuts, as well as stressful living habits, can cause an acidic effect on the body's pH balance. This can be detrimental to fertility as microorganisms such as yeast, bacteria, and viruses thrive in an acidic environment, indirectly affecting the hormonal balance critical to reproduction in both men and women. To promote an alkaline environment, follow these tips:

Drink a warm glass of purified water with lemon first thing in the morning with 2 tbsp apple cider vinegar and wait for 15-20 minutes before consuming anything else. Consume at least six to eight 8-ounce glasses of purified water daily. Incorporate plenty of alkalizing vegetables into your diet.

Enhancing Male Reproductive Health

To improve male fertility, it is important to consume a nutritionally balanced diet and ensure adequate intake of certain nutrients such as zinc, selenium, vitamin B12, omega 3, CoQ10, and vitamin C. These nutrients are essential for the production of healthy and viable sperm. You can obtain these nutrients from various food sources including:

- **Selenium:** Brazil nuts, snapper, cod, halibut, salmon, shrimp, barley, and lean lamb.

- **Vitamin B12:** Lean beef, lean lamb, shrimp, salmon, snapper, and scallops.

- **Zinc:** Lean beef, pork, and lamb, sesame seeds, pumpkin seeds, and shrimp.

- **Vitamin C:** Bell peppers, broccoli, Brussels sprouts, strawberries, oranges, and kiwi.

- **Omega 3:** Mackerel, salmon, herring, oysters, sardines, anchovies, flaxseeds, chia seeds, and walnuts.

- **CoQ10:** Organ meats, fatty fish (trout, mackerel, sardines), beef, broccoli, and tofu.

In addition to following these dietary guidelines, men can also consider other lifestyle changes such as reducing stress, quitting smoking, limiting alcohol consumption, and exercising regularly to further improve their fertility.

Alleviating Anxiety

While dealing with fertility issues, reducing stress may be difficult, but it is necessary as stress is detrimental to fertility. You need to either eliminate stress or learn how to manage it in a healthy way. Here are some methods that you can try:

- **Deep breathing:** breathe into your lower abdomen so that the breath is slow and deep. Try box breathing, also known as four-square breathing, which involves exhaling to a count of four, holding your lungs empty for a four-count, inhaling at the same pace, and holding air in your lungs for a count of four before exhaling and beginning the pattern again.

- **Meditation:** try to meditate for at least 20 minutes every day. Sit in a comfortable, quiet place and concentrate on your breathing while attempting to clear your mind.

- **Yoga:** brilliant for reducing stress and toxins that occur in the body.

- **Weight training:** weight training improves sperm production and reduces stress.

- **Swimming:** burns calories and generates endorphins without putting pressure on joints.

- **Walking:** I call this time on feet! Walking 30- 40 minutes every single day will improve your fertility.

Quit Smoking

To maximize your fertility, it's crucial to steer clear of harmful substances, especially cigarette smoke. Even if you eat healthily and manage your stress levels, smoking will still negatively affect your fertility. Therefore, quitting smoking should be a top priority. Additionally, be mindful of potential toxins in your home and work environment, such as cleaning products and pesticides.

Maintain a Healthy Body Mass Index (BMI)

Maintaining a healthy Body Mass Index (BMI) is also essential for optimal fertility. While being either underweight or overweight can have adverse effects on fertility, research suggests that a BMI between 20 and 24 is the ideal range. So, aim to keep your BMI within this range to boost your chances of conceiving.

Body Mass Index (BMI) is calculated by dividing your weight in pounds by the square of your height in inches and then multiplying by 703. So if you are 125 pounds and are 5 feet, 5 inches (or 65 inches), your BMI = (125 divided by (65 x 65)) x 703 = 21.

Engage in Moderate Physical Activity

Engaging in moderate exercise is highly beneficial for enhancing blood oxygenation and promoting circulation throughout the entire body, including the reproductive region. I recommend a routine of physical activity spanning three to six days each week, which may involve activities like walking, cycling, or swimming, with a minimum duration of 30-40 minutes per session. It's important to avoid intense or strenuous exercise, especially during fertility treatment and maintaining a heart rate at or below 120 beats per minute while exercising. So, while it's encouraged to stay active, it's best to opt for gentler and more relaxed forms of exercise.

Harness the Power of Visualization and Affirmation

Dealing with fertility challenges can be a daunting and exhausting experience. That's why it's crucial to take care of yourself and get enough rest. Visualization is a powerful healing technique that can help you achieve your desired outcome or promote healing in your body. You can try looking for fertility-related CDs or websites that offer guided imagery exercises.

One example is Julia Indichova's Fertile Heart Imagery program, which you can find on her website. Sarah Blondin's guided heart-minded meditations from Insight Timer, Apple Music, and Spotify are also soothing.

Affirmations can also help you stay focused on positive results and improve your overall outlook.

Making changes to your lifestyle and diet can be challenging, but it's important to give yourself time to adjust and celebrate the progress you make. Embrace healthy eating habits and take care of your body and mind. Remember that this is a time to prioritize self-care and give yourself the attention you deserve.

Lead Exposure

Exposure to lead can have detrimental effects on fertility. Lead is a toxic heavy metal that, when absorbed into the body, can disrupt various physiological processes. In both men and women, lead exposure can lead to reduced fertility by impairing the quality and quantity of sperm and eggs. In men, it can lower sperm count, motility, and morphology, making it more challenging to achieve pregnancy. In women, lead can interfere with the menstrual cycle, disrupt hormone production, and increase the risk of miscarriage. Furthermore, lead exposure during pregnancy can harm the developing fetus, potentially leading to birth defects or developmental issues.

Mercury Exposure

Mercury exposure is nearly ubiquitous, present in common household items (electrical parts, pesticides, and certain cosmetics) and fish we consume (tuna and shark). Amalgam fillings are a debated mercury source, as some argue they may start leaking after some years. If you think elevated mercury levels might be affecting your fertility, consult a kinesiologist who employs muscle tests in their diagnostic approach to pinpoint issues.

Cleaning Supplies

Numerous cleaning solutions should be dodged by all, particularly couples attempting conception. Fortunately, eco-friendly alternatives are widely available nowadays, providing a toxin-free method for maintaining a neat living space.

Gardening Supplies

Lawn and garden sprays can pose risks to couples seeking to conceive. Ditch the pesticides and choose a more organic approach to lawn and garden care.

Ecological Contaminants

Our surroundings are teeming with toxins that potentially hinder our reproductive abilities. Prime offenders include xenohormones, synthetic chemicals found in food and our environment that can induce hormonal disruptions, ovary damage (damaged follicles, resulting in diminished progesterone production), and additional fertility issues.

Xenohormones appear in petrochemical-derived pesticides, soap and cosmetic emulsifiers, plastics, and non-organic meat.

Solvents, the most prevalent xenohormone category we encounter regularly, are typically discovered in adhesives, dry-cleaned clothing, nail polish, and paint. They can trigger a variety of health complications, such as exhaustion, unease, despondency, cerebral inflammation, fetal harm, and cerebral oxygen deprivation.

Even worse (while attempting to conceive), these pseudo-hormones tend to imitate estrogen behavior in our bodies, resulting in hormonal turmoil by harming the ovaries, lowering progesterone levels, triggering estrogen-sensitive sites, and obstructing the liver's estrogen production capacity. Ultimately, this may cause ovarian cysts to form, further hampering your journey toward parenthood.

When female embryos are exposed to xenobiotics (environmental contaminants that resemble estrogen's chemical influence on the baby's developing tissues), the ovarian follicles are negatively affected and become dysfunctional. Consequently, they fail to undergo ovulation or generate adequate progesterone. Frightening, right? Absolutely! I can't overstate the necessity of reducing contact with these hazardous environmental substances.

Acupuncture and Traditional Chinese Herbal Medicine Guidelines

Acupuncture genuinely helps enhance a woman's ability to conceive! Even Western medical professionals are now recommending acupuncture to patients. Research published in a systemic review and meta-analysis published in the February 2008 issue of the British Medical Journal indicates that acupuncture can increase the chances of getting pregnant for women undergoing IVF treatment by 65%.

Acupuncture and acupressure specialists explain the reason as follows: Acupuncture aids in relaxing the uterus, boosting blood circulation, and forming a thicker endocrine lining, all of which are necessary for improved conception.

The Essence of Acupuncture

Acupuncture involves more than simply poking a patient with numerous needles. Having been practiced for millennia in Asia, acupuncture is utilized to exchange electrons within the body's energy pathways to enhance the body's overall efficiency.

What are Energy Pathways and How do they Impact Fertility

Energy pathways, or meridians, are lines of energy coursing through our bodies. They exhibit a distinct influence on each of the body's systems, including the reproductive system. Meridians are lines of energy running through the body.

They have a very unique effect on each of the body's systems, including the reproductive system.

What's the link between meridians and fertility? To address this, we must first delve into the formation of meridians and their relationship with bodily systems. As an embryo grows in a woman's uterus, its cells continuously divide. As they cluster, they generate distinct lines that differentiate and connect similar cell groups. These clusters eventually become the body's internal organs.

Remarkably, these "folds" persist after birth, linking all cell groups via "meridian energy pathways." This might clarify why acupoints on the arms or feet can impact organs like the kidneys or ovaries. When electrical energy faces resistance, it can build up, causing issues. Acupuncture serves as an effective method to alleviate this tension and restore adequate energy flow.

Extraordinary Meridians (Vessels)

The Extraordinary Meridians are hormone regulators, aligned with the Western endocrine system which makes them especially important for supporting the different phases of the menstrual cycle. Four extraordinary vessels that are associated with reproduction are the Penetrating Vessel (Chong Mai), Conception Vessel (Ren Mai), Governing Vessel (Du Mai) and Girdle Vessel (Dai Mai).

The Penetrating Vessel (Chong Mai)

This meridian governs a woman's hormonal cycles, managing Yin and Yang energies within the body. The Chong Mai is called the "Sea of Blood" which is why it is so important for treating any gynecological issues as it plays a key role in maintaining a healthy period.

The Conception Vessel (Ren Mai)

The Conception Vessel controls the body's Yin meridians, responsible for generating estrogen that is essential for the female system to function correctly. This meridian is all about nurturing, containing, and holding.

The Governing Vessel (Du Mai)

The Governing Vessel supervises the production of Yang hormones, such as progesterone and testosterone. The Governing Vessel nourishes the Yang channels which is why it is known as "The Sea of Yang."

The Girdle Vessel (Dai Mai)

This meridian encircles the body horizontally around the waist and connects the Penetrating and Conception meridians and consolidates all the meridians that run vertically, helping prevent vaginal leakage and miscarriage.

How Acupuncture Supports Fertility

Firstly, acupuncture needles prompt endorphin production, harmonize the body's energies, and maintain optimal organ function. Additionally, the pressure applied by the acupuncture needle generates a micro-electric current within the body, triggering the release of prostaglandins into the bloodstream and signaling the hypothalamus to regulate hormones.

Acupuncture's stimulation of the pituitary gland can also benefit men, enhancing sperm concentration, volume, and motility. In the world of acupuncture, it's crucial to understand that varied points yield varied results. Selecting a skilled practitioner to address your unique concerns is key to successful treatment.

The Role of Acupuncture in Improving Pelvic Blood Circulation and its Significance

While most individuals recognize the significance of ovulation for conception, few grasp the crucial part pelvic blood circulation plays in maintaining a regular menstrual cycle and healthy ovaries. Both the uterus and ovaries need sufficient blood supply to function optimally.

Without it, the required environment for egg fertilization and implantation to create a baby cannot be formed, hindering pregnancy.

Studies have revealed that acupuncture can ease uterine artery constriction, enhance blood circulation to reproductive organs, and consequently boost a woman's probability of conceiving. Note: Presently, acupuncture is the sole verified method to directly improve vascular response!

Benefits of Acupressure

Acupressure and acupuncture can aid in conception in two crucial ways.

1. By suppressing the sympathetic nervous system.
2. By augmenting the efficacy of other medical approaches.

The body consists of a network of responses and feedback mechanisms. Like a domino effect, applying pressure to certain points or meridians can stimulate blood flow and relay signals to specific body areas to boost fertility.

While acupuncture needles might provide the most benefits for many, some people are too apprehensive about the process and prefer the less invasive acupressure therapy.

Acupressure employs similar principles but without needles.

Another advantage of acupressure is that, with proper guidance and knowledge of the relevant points, you can often self-administer the treatment.

Moxa Therapy

Moxa heat therapy, also known as moxibustion, has been recognized for its potential benefits in enhancing fertility. This traditional Chinese medicine technique involves the burning of dried mugwort (Artemisia vulgaris) near specific acupuncture points, which generates a gentle warmth that permeates the body. By stimulating these points, moxibustion aims to regulate the flow of Qi (life force energy) and balance the body's Yin and Yang forces, which are integral for optimal reproductive health.

One of the primary reasons moxa heat therapy is considered beneficial for fertility is its ability to improve blood circulation, particularly in the pelvic region. Improved blood flow to the reproductive organs fosters a healthier environment for egg production, implantation, and overall uterine health. In addition, moxibustion may help alleviate stress and anxiety often associated with fertility struggles, promoting relaxation and a positive state of mind conducive to conception.

Laser Therapy

Radiance emitted by a compact, scarlet-hued light wand is capable of activating acupressure points just like traditional acupuncture needles. Astonishing as it may seem, these luminous beams can genuinely pierce skin layers, enhancing mitochondrial activity and ATP (energy) of older eggs, increasing blood flow, regulating inflammation, reducing oxidative damage, and reducing pain. Optimal outcomes arise when pressing the gleaming tip against the body's acupressure points for 20-30 seconds.

Magnetic Therapy

Magnetic therapy, a form of alternative medicine, has been explored as a potential adjunct treatment for fertility issues. While scientific evidence remains inconclusive, some individuals have reported benefits in this context. Potential advantages of magnetic therapy for fertility treatment may include:

① **Non-invasive approach:** As a non-pharmacological and non-surgical intervention, magnetic therapy offers a less invasive option for individuals seeking fertility support.

② **Reduced stress:** Proponents of magnetic therapy argue that it can help alleviate stress, which is known to negatively impact fertility. By promoting relaxation and overall well-being, magnetic therapy may indirectly support reproductive health.

③ **Complementary treatment:** Magnetic therapy can be used alongside conventional fertility treatments, potentially enhancing their efficacy or mitigating side effects.

④ **Minimal side effects:** When applied appropriately, magnetic therapy typically has few adverse effects, making it a relatively low-risk option for those seeking fertility support.

⑤ **Cost-effective:** In comparison to many conventional fertility treatments, magnetic therapy can be more affordable, making it a more accessible option for a wider range of individuals.

Additional Guidelines to Support Fertility

Acupressure

Much has been said about the significance of readying your body for conception. You've acquired knowledge on living a healthier life and employing various Chinese medicine practices to boost your likelihood of becoming pregnant. As you now comprehend the connection between your inner energies and your capacity to conceive, it's crucial to nourish all your organs and strengthen your vital energy. Acupressure and Qi Gong exercises are two excellent methods to achieve this.

Qi Gong

What makes acupressure and Qi Gong exercises essential for successful conception? Chinese wisdom teaches that stress in a woman can cause tension in her abdomen (the core of her internal energy), leading to a redirection of her vital energy away from her reproductive organs. This may severely impair her ability to have a child.

For ages, Chinese medicine has been grounded in the Taoist concept of "ancient wisdom."

This fundamental philosophy originates from an age-old tale in which a wise elder from the mountains advised a young man to empty his cup to make space for the knowledge the elder would share. The young man refused, clinging to his worries and burdens, never experiencing the liberation that true knowledge brings.

This philosophy continues to guide Eastern medicine today, as practitioners seek ways to empty their patients' cups to uncover the internal remedy for their ailments. Acupressure and Qi Gong exercises are contemporary applications of this ancient wisdom, developed over time to redirect energy and blood circulation toward the organs that require it most, and to reestablish internal equilibrium in a woman, preparing her body to accommodate and nurture a pregnancy.

Lower Disphragmatic Breathing

To fully unblock your body's airways, it's crucial to become proficient in diaphragmatic breathing. This technique enables total relaxation and promotes rest, digestion, and circulation, and shifts the body from the 'fight or flight' response to a more peaceful and relaxed state. Close your eyes and focus on your breath. Place your hands on your lower abdomen. As you inhale feel your abdomen rise and expand. As you exhale, feel your abdomen contract, gently drawing towards the spine. Continue this lower diaphragmatic breathing for 5 to 10 minutes.

The Uterine Repositioning

Maintaining a robust and well-positioned uterus is vital for a healthy pregnancy. Regrettably, numerous women don't realize that their uterus might be improperly aligned. Various factors can cause your uterus to shift lower than its ideal location: giving birth, poor nutrition, and excessive standing.

Fortunately, this uterine repositioning offers an effortless solution. With this straightforward method, most women can realign their uterus to its optimal position within the body, fortifying it for future tasks.

When you next visit the restroom to urinate, start preparing your uterus for repositioning by contracting forcefully to expel your urine.

Next, engage your pelvic floor muscles to halt the flow (this action is similar to performing a Kegel). Repeat this several times during urination. You are now prepared to reposition your uterus.

Initiate by placing your hands atop your pubic bone. Shift your fingertips just above this bone and firmly press toward your spine. Once you're unable to press further toward your spine, you'll know you've reached the area directly beneath your uterus. At this point, use your fingers to gently elevate your uterus toward your navel. Maintain this posture for a minimum of 30 seconds, then relax.

Potent Qi Gong Practices

Movement is the core of existence. Neglecting to provide your body with the necessary physical activity leads to stagnant Qi, resulting in severe obstructions in every organ. Men, in particular, may experience Qi shortages impacting their fertility, necessitating additional attention to maintaining an active lifestyle.

Naturally, not all forms of exercise or activity promote fertility for both men and women. That's why I have incorporated these vital Qi Gong practices into this book. Qi Gong, akin to Tai Chi, focuses on blood and energy flow throughout the body to boost fertility for both genders. Qi Gong is simpler to learn than Tai Chi and requires less space, making it more accessible for most couples.

Swing Arms

This simple movement enhances circulation, releases tension in the neck and shoulders, and flushes your lymphatic system. Just 6 minutes of this powerful technique has wonderful benefits for your health and fertility. Stand with your feet shoulder-width apart. Your harms should be hanging loosely at your sides. Swing your arms forward to the height of your shoulders and let them swing backward past your hips like a pendulum.

Dan Tien Tapping

This effective fertility-enhancing technique should not be performed post-ovulation, as it may hinder the implantation of a fertilized egg. However, feel free to practice during the first half of your cycle (between the initial day of your period and up to 24 hours before ovulation). To execute this exercise:

• Fully relax your arms, allowing them to swing naturally from side to side until your right-hand strikes your navel area simultaneously as your left hand hits the Life Gateway point on your spine.
• Complete 35 repetitions on each side.

Ensuring Sufficient Sperm, and Intimacy Techniques

Semen Volume: Increase it Before Attempting Pregnancy

Various actions can be taken by a man to enhance his semen volume before his partner's fertile window, ensuring optimal conditions during conception attempts. This entails abstaining from ejaculation for 3-5 days. In this period, engaging in specific yoga exercises or Tantric intimacy techniques can further augment semen production. Engaging in multiple rounds of prolonged arousal, without climax, can improve both semen quantity and quality.

However, boosting semen volume during the incorrect phase of the menstrual cycle will not benefit your baby-making endeavors. While it is feasible to start increasing semen production and motility immediately, it is crucial to initiate 3-5 days before anticipated ovulation. One effective method is practicing oral stimulation, bringing the man close to climax several times within an hour.

Intimacy Positions, Timing, and Vital Suggestions

Do not treat intimacy as a duty, particularly when attempting to conceive. For instance, when one partner is uninterested or fatigued, this can often happen. Nevertheless, this shouldn't deter you from maintaining passion and excitement in your relationship. Sustaining love between partners can help alleviate stress.

The timing of intercourse is crucial for maximizing fertility. It should be planned just before ovulation. Many women can intuitively sense impending ovulation.

However, there are typical indicators to observe, or an ovulation prediction kit can be purchased from a local store.

Happiness has been shown to enhance sperm quality during intimacy. As a result, avoid rushing the process. Slow down and engage in a sensual session of arousal, ensuring both partners are stimulated before penetration. This increases the secretions that comprise semen, subsequently raising ejaculate volume.

Do Not Refrain from Intimacy for Over 3 Days

Refraining from intimacy for more than 3 days to conserve semen is not advised. Engaging in intimacy at least once every 5 days when not attempting to conceive is recommended to ensure fresh and healthy sperm when conception is desired. Penetrative intercourse isn't necessary; ejaculation can be assisted by other means.

During the pre-ovulation phase, frequent intercourse is recommended, ideally daily. This enables plenty of waiting sperm to await the egg in the cervix as it is released. If daily intercourse is not feasible or negatively impacts sperm count, schedule it every other day. This guideline is flexible, and you can adapt it to your preferences. If daily intimacy suits you, embrace it.

Is Timing Significant

Surprisingly, weather can impact sperm production. Cold weather promotes peak sperm production, making winter a preferable time to attempt conception than summer. The sperm count is also higher in the morning than at any other time. Although no specific time or season has been proven superior for conception, this information may be helpful if sperm count is a concern.

Lubrication

Do you rely on store-bought lubricants during intimacy? This could hinder conception. Your body's natural lubrication is best when attempting to conceive. The vagina is typically acidic, while sperm require alkaline conditions. During ovulation, the vagina adapts to accommodate sperm, producing alkaline discharge with an egg-white consistency.

This change enables sperm to traverse the cervix. Enhancing conception chances requires utilizing natural lubrication, which means increasing foreplay to stimulate lubrication and create a sperm-friendly environment.

If natural lubrication is insufficient, continue reading for guidance on selecting appropriate lubricants. Many commercial options have excessively high pH levels, making them too acidic for sperm. Avoid these, including KY Jelly, baby oil, and Vaseline. Canola oil and pharmaceutical-grade mineral oil are more sperm-friendly but remain in a grey area, so their use is not advised.

Pre-Seed is the only sperm-friendly commercial lubricant. It prevents sperm from dying prematurely and has helped many women struggling with lubrication to conceive. Rest assured that you won't have to suffer due to a lack of suitable commercial lubricants when trying to conceive. Homemade options, such as egg white, are also viable.

Egg whites are an excellent choice, often used in laboratories to store sperm. To try this alternative, crack an egg and use the egg white immediately as you would a commercial lubricant.

If refrigerated, let it warm to room temperature first. However, be aware that egg whites can potentially contain traces of salmonella, which may cause infection, although the risk is minimal.

Beware of Soap and Saliva

Soap is detrimental to sperm, so ensure your hands are well-rinsed after washing. Saliva can also be lethal to sperm, particularly sperm motility, making it unwise to use it as a lubricant during sex when attempting to conceive.

Position Choices

It may sound surprising, but specific sexual positions can enhance your probability of conceiving. Consequently, understanding the ideal positions and post-intercourse practices can boost your likelihood of conception. Gravity is an ally! Keep this in mind as you experiment with various positions, as it can expedite your journey toward pregnancy.

Opt for a position that allows deep penetration and cervix contact while minimizing fluid leakage. Penetration from behind ("doggy style") has long been considered one of the most effective positions for conception. The side-by-side stance and man-on-top missionary pose are also excellent options.

To reduce leakage, exercise some restraint. Instead of immediately withdrawing after intercourse, maintain the presence of your partner's penis inside for an extended period post-ejaculation. This action obstructs the cervix entrance, retaining the semen and concentrating it within the cervix for an extended duration.

After intercourse, elevate your hips for approximately 20 to 30 minutes. Use a pillow for support by positioning it under your buttocks. This practice encourages sperm to travel in the correct direction, aided by gravity.

A Retroverted/Tilted Uterus May Pose a Challenge

Nonetheless, it is manageable. If your doctor has informed you of a tilted uterus, don't worry - it will not hinder your conception chances. However, you'll need to modify the advice provided earlier. For those with a tilted uterus, the optimal position is a rear entry. Additionally, after intercourse, lie on your stomach instead of your back, with a pillow placed under your hips.

Chapter 7

The Holistic Approach to Improving Fertility for Women Over 40

How Mind, Body, and Stress Affect Your Pregnancy

It is of the utmost importance that you listen to your body and its signs or signals. Your body tends to indicate to you exactly what is going on and if you are in tune with it, you should know. There are numerous stories of women who are trying to conceive and know within a month or two that something is wrong only to be told by their doctors to keep on trying.

Eventually, after a year or two of continuous disappointment, the doctors finally agree that something is amiss and then proceed to carry out long and drawn-out tests to get to the root of the matter. A lot of time would have been saved if the doctors had listened to the woman's instinct.

Now is the best time to listen to your body and the first step is to look out for ovulation signs so you can act accordingly. Having sex at the right time counts and this can be achieved by watching out for telling signs such as:

• Tender breasts, headaches, and irritability
• More elastic cervical mucus
• A sudden spike in body temperature of at least 0.5 to 1 degree for a period of 3 consecutive days
• One-sided, lower abdominal pain is commonly known as "mittelschmerz" which is German for "middle pain"

Track Your Fertility

Once you have mastered how to detect ovulation, you will need to keep a diary of your fertility signs and symptoms to track and better predict it as time goes on. It might sound difficult and complicated but a fertility chart or mobile app is an easy way to record your information.

All you have to do is write down what you're feeling or type it up on your digital devices. The important thing is to have a record that you can refer to. This will help you be more accurate in predicting ovulation and your period.

Modern Fertility Tools

Knowing when you ovulate can help you plan for sex at the right time and improve your chance of getting pregnant.

Ovulation Kits

These kits can be obtained from various drugstores and while they can be expensive, they offer a lot of value in the predictions of ovulation. They predict ovulation by measuring the quality of Luteinizing Hormone (LH) from your urine.

The levels of this hormone typically rises 24 to 36 hours before ovulation and these tests can correctly predict when you are most likely to ovulate month to month.

There are some limitations to these tests. Some women usually have high LH consistently so for them the results will always be positive. This is also a similar case for women with polycystic ovary syndrome (PCOS) and premature ovarian failure (POF). These kits can also be a little difficult to read and understand.

Saliva Testing

One of the most recent advancements in the field of ovulation testing involves the utilization of saliva testing as a method to track a woman's fertile window.

Specifically, it focuses on the rise in estrogen levels that typically precedes ovulation. When estrogen levels surge, it can have a fascinating and observable effect on the properties of dried saliva.

This phenomenon gives rise to a distinctive and intriguing pattern, often described as resembling delicate fern-like structures when viewed under a microscope.

Home Sperm Testing

As we have discussed multiple times now, fertility issues aren't tied to women alone. Men also play a role. You can obtain a very comprehensive semen analysis in a clinic but you also have the option of doing a quick sperm test at home and you can at least have an idea if you have a sperm count issue.

Monitor Your Fertility

If you wish to make use of a more advanced method to determine fertility, a fertility monitor might be the answer. These monitors have the ability to test to estrogen and LH levels on a daily basis and you can use a small computer to monitor and track your results. Fertility monitors can also be used when you are on fertility meds. One major advantage of these kits is that they can be used for women with erratic and unpredictable cycles.

The Two-Week Wait

Waiting can be a very difficult thing especially when a lot of hope and dreams hinge on your ability to get pregnant. Since you cannot accurately predict pregnancy until at least two weeks after conception, a lot of couples are quite nervous in those two weeks when they have to wait and see. How best to get through this two-week window without going crazy is very valuable information.

Some tips to support you during this time:

① **Get busy with something else:** embark on a new project that can take your mind off everything.

② **Limit your thoughts and conversations about and around babies during this time**. This might be hard but constantly thinking about babies will make this two-week window a lot harder to get through.

③ **Enjoy yourself, have some fun, and explore other things.** Visit family and friends and go to new places. Have a date night!

④ **Have sex just for the sake of it.** A lot of couples trying to get pregnant tend to fall into a cycle where sex just becomes a means to an end and that end is getting pregnant. This takes out the fun. When you eventually become parents, you will have a lot less time to have sex so you best enjoy yourself while you can.

Exercise for Improved Fertility

There are a lot of advantages to exercising properly for both men and women especially when you are trying to conceive. Various activities such as strengthening your body, oxygenating tissues, and detoxification help to alleviate the stress levels that can inhibit conception.

Too much exercise can also be counterproductive and detrimental because they deplete Yin and estrogen levels in the body. When you focus too much energy on your skeletal system, it can have a negative impact on your reproductive system so you have to be smart about your exercise routine.

Stress is not Conducive to Pregnancy

A lot of things can be better accomplished if you just relax. This can be easier said than done but the fact still remains. Stress can be a major hindrance to your success in conception. It is sometimes referred to as the fertility killer and can have a very negative impact on your overall well-being.

Constantly having your body in a fight or flight mode inhibits your reproductive system from operating properly. Stress redirects blood flow away from the areas where you need it the most for conception. This can prevent your body from producing the right amount of hormones.

Get Enough Sleep

There are so many benefits of sleep to our overall well-being and health but what does it do to our fertility? There is really no balance in your body if you aren't getting the right amount of sleep. You have to ensure you get a good 8 hours of sleep every night and take time throughout the day to rest and meditate. This puts your body in the perfect balance.

Dealing with Overwhelm

Being diagnosed with infertility can be an extremely confronting and challenging experience. People often talk about the 'roller coaster', or ups and downs of emotions associated with infertility. It is extremely normal for you and your partner to feel stressed about what is often considered a life crisis. However, there are some important points to keep in mind when you are feeling overwhelmed:

• You are not the only one going through this. Up to one in six couples worldwide have difficulty conceiving in the first 12 months of trying and going through the same processes as you with successful results.

• Everyone feels strong and mixed emotions about what they are experiencing. It is normal to feel shock, anger, anxiety, fear, sadness, guilt, and many other emotions.
• There are many coping techniques and numerous avenues of support, which you can use to assist you when you need it.

Learn to Manage Stress

Learning to manage your stress is an important step toward making sure that you and your partner achieve your goal of becoming parents. This book looks at some of the common emotions that you may experience when confronted with infertility and also includes some techniques and tools for managing them. There are certain stages or situations, which are commonly described as being more difficult and we will discuss some ways to help you cope during those tough times.

Everyone reacts to the diagnosis of infertility differently and it is normal to ask 'Why me?' and to feel sad, angry, worried, or just totally shocked. However, for most people, it is the strength of the emotional impact that often takes them by surprise.

In reaction to a diagnosis of infertility, you may experience a number of emotions such as:

Shock, surprise, or denial – a sense that the diagnosis is not really true. This can also be described as feeling numb or not knowing what to do.

Anger and frustration – this can be expressed as 'Why is this happening to me?' or feeling angry at others.

Anxiety, fear, or panic – all thoughts are very confused.

Isolation – feeling different from others and feeling out of touch with your partner.

Sense of loss – there are many aspects of grief covering loss of pregnancy, loss of motherhood, and fatherhood. These can continue through all stages of infertility.

The way you react and cope with your emotions will be influenced by many things such as:

• how do you interpret the situation
• how you have responded to past stresses
• other events that are also happening in your life
• what type and level of support do you have around you

While all of your emotions are perfectly normal in the face of such a major life crisis, it is important that you do not let these feelings go on for too long or allow them to negatively affect how you manage and cope with everyday life. Learning to recognize and manage your emotional feelings about infertility is as crucial as looking after yourself physically.

You will also need to be aware that there may come a time when these emotions get out of hand and become potentially dangerous. If you are feeling extremely sad or hopeless for more than a couple of weeks and your feelings are interfering with your usual daily activities, you may be suffering from depression and will need to seek help from a healthcare professional.

Hormonal Changes

In addition to dealing with feelings of uncertainty and trepidation, as well as hope, you will be dealing with the impact of hormonal changes on your body. Responses to the medications used to stimulate the ovaries during IVF vary enormously.

Some women have no symptoms while others feel emotional and much more prone to tears, anxiety, and irritability. Others feel uncomfortable with bloating, headaches, tiredness, and other symptoms.

While you cannot help the way you feel, you may be able to find a way to better manage your feelings and reactions during these times.

Positive Reappraisal Technique

The Positive Reappraisal Technique can help you manage some of the negative emotions that are associated with the diagnosis of infertility.

All situations involve some good and some bad aspects and the aspects we pay attention to often determine how we feel. Thinking more about the positive points of a difficult situation and dwelling less on problems or uncertainties for the future helps people feel better.

This does not mean we should pretend that everything is wonderful when we do not feel it is or think that we will definitely get pregnant when we feel unsure. What it does mean is that you are choosing to remind yourself that even very challenging situations have some positive elements.

Remember that it will take time for you to come to terms with your emotions, and you will most likely have your good days and bad days. Choose a few statements from those below that will help you cope better each day. Try to make the time to rest and recuperate every day, as you will be better able to manage your emotions when you are not feeling tired.

The Positive Reappraisal Technique is a cognitive-behavioral coping strategy aimed at helping individuals manage stress, negative emotions, and challenging situations by reframing their perspective and finding positive aspects of the experience.

This technique is rooted in the idea that our thoughts and interpretations of events are largely influenced by our emotional responses, and by changing our perspective, we can change how we feel.

Here are the main steps to practice the Positive Reappraisal Technique:

① **Identify the situation:** Begin by acknowledging the event or situation that is causing you distress or negative emotions. Be specific and honest with yourself about your feelings.

② **Analyze your thoughts:** Reflect on your thoughts and beliefs about the situation. Identify any negative or irrational thoughts that may be contributing to your emotional response.

③ **Challenge negative thoughts:** Question the accuracy and validity of your negative thoughts. Consider alternative perspectives or explanations for the situation, and evaluate if there is any evidence to support the negative thought.

④ **Reframe the situation:** Develop a new, more positive perspective on the situation by focusing on the potential benefits, opportunities for growth, or lessons that can be learned. This may involve finding a silver lining, recognizing your own resilience or strengths, or acknowledging the support of others.

⑤ **Embrace the new perspective:** Accept and internalize the new, more positive perspective, and allow it to influence your emotional response to the situation. This may involve using positive affirmations, visualizing the positive aspects, or discussing your new perspective with others.

Practicing the Positive Reappraisal Technique regularly can help women build resilience, reduce stress, and enhance overall well-being by promoting a more adaptive and optimistic mindset.

Communicating with Your Partner

Good communication is essential in all relationships but this can be strained when you are undergoing IVF or other procedures. It can be hard to talk about something that is so painful, and often we don't mean the angry or hurtful things that we say.

A partner may be grieving in his or her own way which isn't understood by the other partner. We often think that our partner should know how we are feeling or be able to 'read our mind'. It is unfair to assume this if you haven't talked about it. Communication usually has to be worked on. It may be helpful to write down feelings and show these to each other, or make an extra effort to find time to talk. Sometimes going away for a few days together can help.

Handling Emotions and Intimacy

It may be difficult to have spontaneous loving sex when there is so much intimate medical intervention going on.

Sometimes it is better not to worry about sex for a while. It is important, however, to take the time to enjoy some intimate moments, such as cuddling and holding hands.

For others, it may be comforting to have an intimate relationship when everything else seems out of control. Again, talk about fears and feelings – this will help both of you to work out the best solution.

When one partner has an identified fertility problem it can lead to feelings of inadequacy and inequality in the relationship. It helps if partners tackle the problem together, for example going to appointments and talking afterward about what was discussed. Approach the situation as 'our problem', and something to work on together.

Men and women deal with emotions and solve problems differently. You both may care just as deeply about becoming a parent, but express it in different ways. Women tend to confront a problem directly by talking things out. They seem naturally to be able to share feelings, especially with other women.

On the other hand, men find it less natural to share their feelings and try to work out things themselves. They are often accused of trivializing the issue with a "she'll be right mate" attitude or bottling up their feelings. Being aware of these differences can help you avoid misunderstandings and allow you to tackle the challenges as a team.

Despite the strain, most couples who have been through fertility treatment say they're brought closer by the experience and their relationship is stronger at the end.

You'll find it helps to:

• Decide on how you want to communicate and support each other.

• Draw up a plan for the future. It helps to put things in perspective and focus on what's important should you need to make difficult decisions.

• Don't allow fertility to rule your life. Instead, if there's something you need to discuss, set aside a specific time and give the venue some thought. A walk in the park may be less intense than a fixed table for two.

• During conversations try to avoid 'blaming' statements such as 'you always' or 'you never'.

• Put a conscious effort into planning something fun where you don't need to talk about your fertility. It's important to create some balance in your life.

Importance of Open Dialogue

Discussing fertility issues with family members and friends may be uncomfortable, but expressing how you feel may help you release your stress. It's important that you reach out for support.

Infertility is a sensitive subject and many people may not know how to react. Even family members who are aware of your situation can often say the wrong thing.

Guide the conversation and help them avoid topics that may be hurtful or make you feel uncomfortable. Feel free to say you're not in the mood for a heavy chat and ask what's new with them.

It may help if you can talk to your friends and family about the role they can play. Let your friends know how they can support you and give them some detail about what you need, eg, "When I call you and I'm crying, I need you to listen to me. You don't have to give me advice or try to fix anything or even say something earth-shattering just need you to be there for me."

Importance of Open Dialogue

Some friends may be good listeners. Others may be top of your list with whom to have fun when you are feeling down. Think of what you expect from your support network and let them know.

It can be hard to be happy for others who are having babies, and it can seem that everyone around you is pregnant or pushing prams. Keep in mind that it is perfectly normal to feel distressed at others' pregnancies and births. You are not a bad person and this experience will one day be behind you.

Calming Anxiety

Some strategies for calming your anxiety include explaining your situation; not visiting the maternity hospital but visiting when they are back home and don't have others around; and avoiding situations where there may be many young children. If you really feel you have to attend a family event, for example, your sister's baby's christening, then stay for half an hour and leave quietly.

Explain to your sister and other close family members beforehand that this is what is going to happen and ask them to respect your feelings.

Loss of a pregnancy is always hard but it is even more difficult when it has taken so much time and treatment to fall pregnant. It is hard to have hope that pregnancy will happen again. Usual supports may not have been told, so they are not approached for help. Some people withdraw and are private in their grief. Others reach out to friends to discuss their painful loss over and over again.

Some people deal with intense feelings by becoming very busy. Others become very rational and appear able to cope by denying the depth of their pain.

You may feel surprised and guilty that you are not joyful about your pregnancy. You may be fearing that it may not continue could make it hard to relax and enjoy.

Talking about these fears and having reliable support people can be helpful. Stopping treatment is also a time of mixed emotions. Most know when it is time to stop and seek relief from the constant procedures and disappointments. You may decide to stop because you are exhausted with it all. It is important to realize that it will take time to accept that you won't have children from this treatment and that sadness and anger are normal.

It may also be just as hard to realize that you may never know why it didn't work. With the mixed emotions of relief and sadness, there is also the realization that the time of being in limbo has stopped and that it is now possible to take back control.

Understanding Stress and Anxiety in Women Over 40

Stress and anxiety are common experiences that can significantly impact women's health, particularly in relation to fertility. For women over 40, the challenges of fertility are often compounded by societal pressures and personal concerns. Traditional Chinese Medicine (TCM) offers a holistic approach to understanding and addressing these issues, helping women navigate the complex interplay of stress, anxiety, and fertility.

The Connection Between Stress, Anxiety, and Fertility

Research has shown that stress and anxiety can negatively impact fertility in women of all ages. High levels of stress hormones, such as cortisol, can interfere with the delicate balance of hormones necessary for ovulation and conception. In women over 40, age-related declines in fertility make it even more critical to address these factors.

Traditional Chinese Medicine and Stress Reduction

Traditional Chinese Medicine has long recognized the importance of managing stress and anxiety to maintain overall health and well-being. TCM views the body as a network of interconnected systems, with stress and anxiety capable of causing imbalances that can impact fertility. Key TCM concepts relevant to stress, anxiety, and fertility include:

① **Qi (vital energy):** In TCM, the flow of Qi through the body is essential for maintaining health. Stress and anxiety can obstruct the flow of Qi, leading to imbalances that can affect fertility.

② **Yin and Yang:** These opposing forces represent balance and harmony in the body. Excessive stress and anxiety can disrupt the equilibrium between Yin and Yang, causing fertility issues.

③ **The Five Elements:** TCM associates specific organs with each of the five elements (wood, fire, earth, metal, and water). Stress and anxiety can disrupt the harmony of these elements, leading to fertility challenges

TCM Treatments for Stress, Anxiety, and Fertility

Traditional Chinese Medicine offers a variety of treatments to address stress, anxiety, and fertility issues in women over 40. Some common TCM approaches include:

① **Acupuncture:** This ancient practice involves the insertion of thin needles at specific points on the body to regulate the flow of Qi and restore balance. Acupuncture has been shown to reduce stress, anxiety, and improve fertility outcomes in some cases.

② **Herbal Medicine:** TCM practitioners may prescribe customized herbal formulas to address specific imbalances and support fertility. These formulas often include herbs known for their calming and stress-reducing properties, such as jujube (Da Zao), Chinese peony (Bai Shao), and licorice root (Gan Cao).

③ **Diet and Nutrition:** A balanced diet is essential for optimal fertility. TCM emphasizes the importance of consuming foods that nourish and support the body, particularly those that align with an individual's unique constitution.

④ **Mind-Body Practices:** TCM encourages practices like Tai Chi, Qi Gong, and meditation to cultivate inner peace and promote a healthy flow of Qi. These practices can help to reduce stress and anxiety, improving overall wellbeing and fertility

For women over 40, understanding the relationship between stress, anxiety, and fertility is essential for optimizing reproductive health. Traditional Chinese Medicine offers a holistic and integrative approach to addressing these concerns, supporting the body's innate ability to find balance and achieve overall wellbeing.

By incorporating TCM principles and practices into daily life, women can empower themselves to navigate the challenges of fertility with greater ease and confidence.

Understanding Depression in Women Over 40

Some of the warning signs of depression include:

• Helpless or hopeless
• Disappointed
• Indecisive or overwhelmed
• Guilty
• Lack of interest or motivation to perform your normal activities
• Decreased energy and fatigue
• Anxiety
• Irritable, angry, or frustrated
• Mood swings
• Sad or empty
• Inability to concentrate
• Not being able to sleep or sleeping too much
• Significant weight loss or gain
• Extreme anger and resentment
• Uncontrollable emotions
• Social isolation
• Loss of sexual desire or performance
• Persistent thoughts of suicide or death

This can be a time of emotional ups and downs which can be exhausting. It may be hard to understand that something unseen is causing so much distress.

In about 10-15% of couples, a cause for infertility may not be found even after a thorough investigation of both partners. Emotionally, this is the most frustrating and stressful diagnosis of all because there is no cause or management plan to focus on.

It is important that you regularly discuss how you feel with your partner and allow them to offer you their understanding and support and seek help if you see any of the above signs and symptoms. The mainstay of treatment for depression is usually medication but there are therapies such as cognitive behavioral therapy, counseling, psychology, psychotherapy, intensive short-term dynamic psychotherapy (ISDTP), arts and creative therapies, ecotherapy, plant medicine; and complementary and alternative therapies such as acupuncture, kinesiology, hypnosis, meditation, yoga, and eye movement desensitization and reprocessing (EMDR).

This can be a time of emotional ups and downs which can be exhausting. It may be hard to understand that something unseen is causing so much distress.

In about 10-15% of couples, a cause for infertility may not be found even after a thorough investigation of both partners. Emotionally, this is the most frustrating and stressful diagnosis of all because there is no cause or management plan to focus on.

It is important that you regularly discuss how you feel with your partner and allow them to offer you their understanding and support and seek help if you see any of the above signs and symptoms. The mainstay of treatment for depression is usually medication but there are therapies such as cognitive behavioral therapy, counseling, psychology, psychotherapy, intensive short-term dynamic psychotherapy (ISDTP), arts and creative therapies, ecotherapy, plant medicine; and complementary and alternative therapies such as acupuncture, kinesiology, hypnosis, meditation, yoga, and eye movement desensitization and reprocessing (EMDR).

Chapter 8

Enhancing Fertility through Liver Detox: Understanding the Benefits and Effective Techniques

Introduction

This chapter aims to provide you with the necessary knowledge and tools to better understand the connection between liver health and fertility, and to help you implement strategies that can optimize your chances of conception.

The liver is a vital organ, and its role in maintaining overall health and well-being is well-documented in both Eastern and Western medical practices. We begin with an exploration of the liver organ from both perspectives, offering a holistic view of its significance in our lives.

Delving into the topic of detoxification, I will discuss the rationale behind performing a liver detox for fertility and provide an overview of the process. A step-by-step guide with practical tips on how to do a liver detox specifically for fertility purposes, along with recommendations on the foods to eat during the detox to maximize its effectiveness.

As every individual is unique, I will address questions about the duration of a fertility detox (fertility cleanse) and provide guidance on finding the optimal length for your circumstances.

To further support your liver detox, I will discuss the use of supplements, Chinese herbal medicine, and the specific acupuncture points that can help boost fertility.

Finally, I recognize the importance of mental and emotional well-being in the fertility journey. This chapter concludes with mindfulness techniques and strategies designed to help you cope with the stress and anxiety often associated with fertility issues, enabling you to approach your liver detox with a positive mindset and renewed energy.

Embark on this enlightening journey to enhance your fertility through liver detox and discover a world of possibilities that lie ahead.

The Liver Organ- An East-West Perspective

The liver is one of the most critical organs in the human body, responsible for vital functions such as detoxification, metabolism, blood sugar regulation, and hormone production. In both Western and Traditional Chinese Medicine (TCM) perspectives, maintaining liver health is crucial to overall well-being. This is particularly true for women over 40 trying to conceive, as liver health can directly impact fertility. In this sub-chapter, I will explore the importance of liver health for fertility, the benefits of liver detoxification, and the effective techniques to achieve it from an East-West perspective.

The Liver in Western Medicine

In Western medicine, the liver is considered the body's primary detoxification organ. It filters and eliminates toxins from the bloodstream, processes nutrients, and aids in the production of essential hormones, such as estrogen and progesterone. These hormones regulate menstrual cycles, prepare the body for pregnancy, and maintain a healthy pregnancy.

As women age, their liver's detoxification capacity may decline, leading to hormonal imbalances and a decrease in overall fertility. Women over 40 can improve their chances of conception and maintain a healthy pregnancy by supporting liver health.

The Liver in Traditional Chinese Medicine (TCM)

In TCM, the Liver is believed to play a central role in maintaining a smooth flow of energy, or Qi, throughout the body. The Liver is responsible for storing blood and regulating the volume of blood in circulation, which is essential for nourishing the reproductive system. It also governs the smooth flow of emotions, helping to reduce stress and maintain emotional balance. According to TCM, when the Liver is functioning optimally, the body's Qi flows smoothly, promoting overall health, well-being, and fertility.

In TCM, the Liver is closely related to the Kidney system, which is the primary source of reproductive energy. The health of the Liver and Kidneys directly impacts fertility, particularly in women over 40. A healthy Liver supports the Kidneys, helping to preserve reproductive energy and enhance fertility.

Why Detox for Fertility?

The liver plays a vital role in the menstrual cycle, as it is responsible for breaking down and metabolizing hormones, including estrogen and progesterone.

When the liver becomes congested or imbalanced due to various factors such as poor diet, stress, or exposure to toxins, it can negatively impact fertility. A poorly functioning liver may lead to hormonal imbalances, irregular menstruation, or the stagnation of Qi and blood. Therefore, detoxifying and maintaining a healthy liver is essential for enhancing fertility in women over 40.

Benefits of Liver Detox for Fertility

① **Hormonal Balance:** Liver detoxification can help regulate hormone levels in the body. A healthy liver efficiently breaks down and metabolizes hormones, ensuring that they are adequately utilized and excreted. Detoxifying the liver can help maintain hormonal balance, which is essential for regular ovulation, implantation, and healthy pregnancy.

② **Improved Menstrual Cycle:** A healthy liver promotes regular and healthy menstrual cycles. Detoxifying the liver can help reduce menstrual irregularities, such as painful periods, heavy bleeding, or missed periods, which may impact fertility.

③ **Enhanced Egg Quality:** Liver detoxification can help improve the quality of a woman's eggs by ensuring that the liver efficiently removes toxins and supports proper nutrient absorption. This is especially important for women over 40, as egg quality tends to decline with age.

④ **Reduced Stress:** The liver plays a crucial role in managing stress, as it is responsible for breaking down stress hormones. A healthy liver can help manage stress more effectively, which is essential for overall well-being and fertility.

⑤ **Reduced Inflammation:** Chronic inflammation is linked to various health issues, including fertility problems. A liver detox helps to reduce inflammation in the body by eliminating toxins and promoting a healthy internal environment, which can improve fertility outcomes.

Detoxifying the liver is an essential component of enhancing fertility, particularly for women over 40 who are trying to conceive. Optimizing liver function, hormonal balance, menstrual cycle regularity, egg quality, and stress management can be improved, all of which contribute to increased fertility.

In summary, a liver detox from a Traditional Chinese Medicine perspective can offer significant benefits for women over 40 seeking to improve their fertility.

By implementing a combination of acupuncture, herbal medicine, dietary changes, and stress management techniques, women can optimize their liver function and create a healthier environment for conception.

Effective Techniques for Liver Detoxification

① **Diet:** A healthy diet is crucial for liver health. Women over 40 should focus on consuming nutrient-dense foods like fresh fruits and vegetables, lean proteins, and whole grains. In TCM, it is recommended to include liver-supportive foods, such as dark leafy greens, beets, and goji berries.

② **Herbal remedies:** Certain herbs can help support liver detoxification, such as milk thistle, dandelion root, and turmeric. In TCM, practitioners often recommend herbs like bupleurum (Chai Hu), white peony root (Bai Shao), and licorice root (Gan Can) to help cleanse and support liver function.

③ **Acupuncture:** This ancient practice can help regulate the flow of Qi, support liver health, and enhance fertility. Acupuncture treatments specifically targeting the Liver meridian can help improve liver function and overall well-being.

④ **Stress reduction:** High levels of stress can negatively impact liver function and fertility. Engaging in regular stress-reducing activities, such as meditation, yoga, tai chi, or qi gong, can help support liver health and promote emotional well-being. In TCM, these practices are believed to help maintain a smooth flow of Qi, essential for overall health and fertility.

⑤ **Physical exercise:** Moderate exercise is vital for maintaining liver health and promoting fertility. Regular physical activity can improve circulation, support hormonal balance, and help manage stress. In TCM, practices such as Tai Chi and Qi Gong are particularly beneficial for balancing the liver's energy and maintaining overall well-being.

⑥ **Avoiding toxins:** Reducing exposure to environmental toxins, such as alcohol, tobacco, and chemicals found in household and personal care products, can help support liver detoxification and improve overall health. Opting for organic, non-toxic products can significantly reduce the burden on the liver and enhance fertility.

⑦ **Castor oil packs:** Applying a warm castor oil pack on the liver area can help improve circulation, reduce inflammation, and promote detoxification. This natural remedy has been used for centuries to support liver health and improve fertility.

⑧ **Proper sleep:** Adequate sleep is essential for liver health, as it allows the body to regenerate and detoxify. Ensuring a consistent sleep schedule and practicing good sleep hygiene can help support liver function and overall well-being.

Maintaining liver health is crucial for women over 40 looking to enhance their fertility. By understanding the benefits of liver detoxification from both an East-West perspective, women can implement effective techniques to support liver function and increase their chances of conception.

By embracing a holistic approach that combines dietary changes, herbal remedies, acupuncture, stress reduction, physical exercise, toxin avoidance, and proper sleep, women can improve their overall health and well-being, paving the way for a successful pregnancy.

What Should I Eat When I Do A Liver Detox for Fertility

Dietary Recommendations for a Liver Detox in TCM

When undertaking a liver detox for fertility, it is essential to nourish the body with the right foods that align with TCM principles. The following dietary guidelines can help support liver detoxification and enhance fertility:

1. Consume Foods that Support Liver Qi

To enhance liver function and promote the smooth flow of Qi, include foods that have a positive impact on liver health. Some examples of liver-supportive foods are:

- **Leafy green vegetables:** Spinach, kale, and Swiss chard
- **Cruciferous vegetables:** Broccoli, cauliflower, and Brussels sprouts
- **Fruits:** Berries, apples, and citrus fruits
- **Nuts and seeds:** Walnuts, almonds, and flaxseeds
- **Whole grains:** Brown rice, quinoa, and oats
- **Lean proteins:** Fish, chicken, and tofu

2. Avoid Foods that Stagnate Liver Qi

To support liver detoxification and promote fertility, it is essential to avoid foods that can cause stagnation or impair liver function. These include:

- Fried, greasy, or heavily processed foods
- Excessive consumption of dairy and red meat
- Refined sugars and artificial sweeteners
- Alcohol and excessive caffeine

3. Emphasize Warming Foods

In TCM, the concept of warming and cooling foods is essential for maintaining balance in the body. To support liver detoxification and fertility, focus on incorporating warming foods into your diet, such as:

• Ginger
• Cinnamon
• Fennel
• Sweet potatoes
• Black beans

4. Include Kidney–Nourishing Foods

In TCM, kidney health is closely linked to fertility. To support both liver detoxification and kidney function, consume foods that nourish the kidneys, including:

• Black sesame seeds
• Goji berries
• Walnuts
• Kidney beans
• Salmon

By focusing on a diet rich in liver-supportive, warming, and kidney-nourishing foods, women over 40 can support liver detoxification and improve their chances of conceiving. In addition to these dietary recommendations, it is essential to consult with a TCM practitioner or healthcare provider to ensure that a liver detox plan is tailored to your specific needs and circumstances. As with any health-related endeavor, a balanced and holistic approach is key to enhancing fertility and overall well-being.

How Long Should A Fertility Detox (Fertility Cleanse) Last?

Before determining the appropriate length of a fertility detox, it is essential to understand the primary goal of liver detoxification in TCM.

A fertility detox (fertility cleanse), aims to support and strengthen the liver's function in eliminating toxins and maintaining hormonal balance. There is no one-size-fits-all answer to the question of how long a fertility detox should last, as the duration depends on various factors such as the individual's health, lifestyle, and specific fertility concerns. However, TCM practitioners generally recommend a fertility detox program lasting between 4 to 6 weeks. This timeframe allows for the liver to undergo a thorough cleansing process while also providing ample time for the body to adjust to the changes and restore balance.

During a fertility detox, specific dietary and lifestyle changes are recommended, along with herbal remedies and acupuncture treatments that support liver function and overall reproductive health.

A fertility detox or fertility cleanse is a vital component of TCM for women over 40 who are trying to conceive. A comprehensive fertility detox program includes dietary changes, herbal remedies, acupuncture treatments, and stress management techniques to support liver function, hormonal balance, and overall reproductive health. Consult a TCM practitioner for personalized guidance on the optimal duration and components of a fertility detox tailored to your specific needs.

Chinese Herbal Medicine to Support Liver Detox for Fertility

Chinese Herbal Medicine For Liver Detoxification

Chinese herbal medicine offers a variety of natural, plant-based remedies to support liver detoxification and fertility. These herbs and formulas work together to cleanse the liver, promote the smooth flow of Qi and blood, and nourish the reproductive system. Below are some of the most commonly used herbs and formulas in TCM for liver detoxification:

① **Milk Thistle (Silybum marianum):** Milk thistle is a well-known herb in TCM for its liver-protective and detoxifying properties. It contains a compound called silymarin, which has been shown to support liver function, reduce inflammation, and promote liver cell regeneration. This makes milk thistle an essential herb for women over 40 seeking to cleanse their liver and enhance fertility

② **Bupleurum, Bupleurum chinense (Chai Hu):** Bupleurum is a widely used TCM herb for promoting the smooth flow of Qi and relieving liver stagnation. It is often combined with other herbs in formulas such as Xiao Yao San (Free and Easy Wanderer) or Chai Hu Shu Gan San (Bupleurum and Cyperus Combination) to address various liver-related imbalances that may affect fertility.

③ **Schisandra, Schisandra chinensis (Wu Wei Zi):** Schisandra is a powerful adaptogenic herb that helps support liver function and protect it from toxins. It is commonly used in TCM to enhance fertility by reducing stress, promoting hormonal balance, and improving overall vitality.

④ **Goji Berry, Lycium barbarum (Gou Qi Zi):** Goji berries are considered a nourishing tonic in TCM, offering a range of benefits for women's health, including liver support, immune system enhancement, and increased fertility. They are rich in antioxidants, vitamins, and minerals, which can help to protect and nourish the liver and reproductive system.

⑤ **Angelica sinensis (Dang Gui):** Angelica sinensis, also known as Chinese angelica, is a widely used herb in TCM for nourishing the blood and promoting its circulation. It is particularly beneficial for women's reproductive health, as it can help regulate menstruation, alleviate menstrual pain, and improve overall fertility. By supporting liver detoxification, Dang Gui can help enhance the body's natural ability to eliminate toxins and maintain hormonal balance, making it an essential herb for women over 40 trying to conceive.

⑥ **White Peony Root, Paeonia lactiflora (Bai Shao):** White peony root is a popular TCM herb for regulating menstruation, relieving pain, and improving blood circulation. It also plays a crucial role in liver detoxification by helping to reduce liver stagnation and promote the smooth flow of Qi. White peony root is often used in combination with other herbs, such as Dang Gui and Bupleurum, to enhance its effectiveness in promoting fertility.

⑦ **Rehmannia, Rehmannia glutinosa, (Shu Di Huang):** Rehmannia is a vital herb in TCM for nourishing the blood, replenishing the Yin energy, and supporting Kidney function. The Kidneys and Liver are closely linked in TCM, so by nourishing the Kidneys, Rehmannia can indirectly help support liver detoxification. This herb is particularly beneficial for women over 40 trying to conceive, as it can help address the age-related decline in kidney function and improve overall fertility.

⑧ **Turmeric, Curcuma longa (Jiang Huang):** Turmeric is a common spice with potent antioxidant and anti-inflammatory properties. In TCM, it is often used to help reduce liver inflammation, promote the smooth flow of Qi, and support liver detoxification. By improving liver function and reducing inflammation, turmeric can help enhance fertility in women over 40.

⑨ **Reishi Mushroom, Ganoderma lucidum (Ling Zhi):** Reishi is a medicinal mushroom that has been used for centuries in TCM for its immune-boosting and liver-supporting properties. It can help protect the liver from damage, promotes liver cell rejuvenation, tonifies Qi, and nourishes Blood.

⑩ **Dandelion Root, Taraxacum officinale, (Pu Gong Ying):** Dandelion root is a natural diuretic that helps flush toxins from the liver and kidneys. It also stimulates bile production, which aids in the digestion of fats and the absorption of fat-soluble vitamins necessary for fertility.

Acupuncture Points for Fertility Liver Detox

This sub-chapter focuses on the benefits of liver detoxification for fertility and the effective acupuncture points for achieving this from a Traditional Chinese Medicine perspective.

Acupuncture Points for Fertility Liver Detox

The following acupuncture points are particularly effective for liver detoxification and enhancing fertility:

① **Liver 3 (LV 3, Taichong):** Located on the top of the foot, between the first and second toes, this point is essential for liver detoxification. Stimulating LV 3 helps regulate the flow of Qi, alleviate stress, and improve hormonal balance.

② **Liver 14 (LV 14, Qimen):** Located below the nipple, in the sixth intercostal space, LV 14 helps regulate liver Qi and promotes liver detoxification. This point is particularly useful for addressing hormonal imbalances and menstrual irregularities.

③ **Spleen 6 (SP 6, Sanyinjiao):** Located on the inside of the lower leg, four finger breadths above the ankle bone, SP 6 is a powerful point for promoting blood circulation and nourishing the reproductive system. It is beneficial for women over 40 who are trying to conceive, as it helps improve egg quality and supports a healthy menstrual cycle.

④ **Kidney 3 (KD 3, Taixi):** Located on the inside of the ankle, between the Achilles tendon and the ankle bone, KD 3 is essential for supporting kidney function, which is closely linked to fertility in TCM. Stimulating this point can help improve overall reproductive health and support liver detoxification.

⑤ **Ren 4 (CV 4, Guanyuan):** Located on the midline of the lower abdomen, approximately four finger breadths below the navel, Ren 4 is a crucial point for nourishing the reproductive system and promoting fertility. Stimulating this point can help strengthen the uterus and improve hormonal balance, which is essential for women over 40 trying to conceive. Ren 4 is particularly effective in enhancing liver detoxification and promoting a smoother flow of Qi throughout the body, thereby improving overall reproductive health.

⑥ **Ren 6 (CV 6, Qihai):** Located on the midline of the lower abdomen, approximately 3 finger breadths below the navel, Ren 6 is another powerful acupuncture point for fertility. It helps to regulate and support the liver's function, as well as strengthen the kidney and spleen systems. Stimulating this point can improve overall energy levels and increase the body's ability to detoxify, which is crucial for women over 40 who are trying to conceive.

⑦ **Stomach 36 (ST 36, Zusanli):** Located on the outside of the lower leg, about four finger breadths below the kneecap, one finger breadth from the anterior border of the tibia, ST 36 is a vital point for enhancing overall health and well-being. It helps to strengthen the digestive system, which in turn supports liver detoxification. Moreover, stimulating ST 36 can improveQi and blood circulation, positively impacting fertility and reproductive health

⑧ **Pericardium 6 (PC 6, Neiguan):** Situated on the inside of the forearm between the tendons of palmaris longus and flexi carpi radials, about three finger breadths above the wrist crease, PC 6 is a valuable acupuncture point for alleviating stress and promoting emotional well-being. As stress can negatively impact fertility, stimulating this point can help create a more conducive environment for conception. Furthermore, PC 6 supports liver detoxification by promoting the smooth flow of Qi throughout the body.

⑨ **Gallbladder 34 (GB 34, Yanglingquan):** Positioned on the outside of the lower leg, below the knee, and in front of the fibula head, GB 34 is the influential point for tendons and muscles. By stimulating this point, you can help regulate liver Qi, support liver detoxification, and promote emotional balance. It is particularly beneficial for women over 40 who may be experiencing stress-related fertility issues.

Acupuncture Treatment Considerations

When seeking acupuncture treatment for fertility liver detox, it is essential to work with a licensed and experienced acupuncturist who is familiar with treating fertility issues. The acupuncturist will create a customized treatment plan based on your specific needs and health conditions.

It is also important to remember that acupuncture is most effective when used in conjunction with other TCM modalities, such as herbal medicine, dietary therapy, and lifestyle changes. To fully support liver detoxification and enhance fertility, it is crucial to adopt a holistic approach to your overall well-being.

Acupuncture is an effective and natural method for enhancing fertility through liver detoxification, particularly for women over 40 who are trying to conceive. By stimulating specific acupuncture points, you can help regulate the flow of Qi, improve hormonal balance, and create a more conducive environment for conception. Combined with other TCM treatments and a healthy lifestyle, acupuncture can be an invaluable tool in your journey toward achieving a healthy pregnancy.

Mindfulness Techniques and Strategies to Support a Fertility Liver Detox

Mindfulness techniques have long been used in TCM to facilitate relaxation and reduce stress, which in turn helps to support liver function and overall fertility. Below you will find various mindfulness practices that can aid in enhancing fertility through a liver detox, specifically for women over 40 who are trying to conceive.

1. Mindful Breathing

Mindful breathing is a foundational practice in TCM that involves focusing on one's breath to cultivate awareness, relaxation, and overall well-being. This technique can be particularly helpful for supporting a fertility liver detox as it assists in balancing the body's Qi and promotes liver health.

To practice mindful breathing, find a comfortable seated position and close your eyes. Focus on your natural breath as it flows in and out of your body. As thoughts arise, gently redirect your attention to your breath without judgment. Aim to practice for at least 5-10 minutes daily.

2. Meditation

Meditation is another powerful mindfulness technique that can help to support liver detoxification and enhance fertility. Regular meditation practice has been shown to reduce stress, balance hormones, and promote overall well-being, all of which are essential for optimal liver function.

For women over 40 trying to conceive, consider practicing a fertility-focused meditation. Begin by finding a quiet and comfortable space to sit. Close your eyes and take a few deep breaths to settle your body and mind. Visualize your liver as a source of vibrant, nurturing energy that supports your reproductive system. As you breathe, imagine this energy flowing throughout your body, nourishing your ovaries, uterus, and fallopian tubes. Practice this visualization for 10-20 minutes daily.

3. Yoga

Yoga is a holistic practice that combines physical postures, breathwork, and mindfulness to promote overall health and well-being. Incorporating a gentle yoga practice into your routine can be particularly beneficial for supporting liver detoxification and fertility.

Several yoga poses are known to stimulate the liver and support its detoxification process. These include forward bends, twists, and inversions. Additionally, practicing yoga can help to reduce stress and balance hormones, which are crucial for women in their 40s trying to conceive. Aim to practice yoga 3-5 times per week for optimal benefits.

4. Mindful Eating

The foods we consume can have a significant impact on our liver health and fertility. Adopting a mindful eating approach can help to support liver detoxification and improve overall well-being.

To practice mindful eating, begin by choosing nutrient-dense, liver-supportive foods such as leafy greens, cruciferous vegetables, and lean proteins. As you eat, focus on the flavors, textures, and sensations of each bite. Chew slowly and savor the experience. This mindful approach to eating can help to improve digestion, reduce stress, and support liver function.

5. Emotional Release Techniques

In TCM, the liver is closely associated with the smooth flow of emotions. When emotions become stagnant or suppressed, this can negatively impact liver function and overall fertility. Emotional release techniques, such as journaling, can be an effective way to process and release emotions, supporting liver detoxification and fertility.

Set aside time each day to write about your thoughts and emotions as you journey through the process of enhancing fertility and supporting liver detoxification. This can help to alleviate stress and promote emotional well-being, both of which are essential for optimal liver function and fertility. As you write, allow yourself to explore any fears, anxieties, or frustrations that may arise without judgment. By giving yourself permission to express and release these emotions, you can create space for healing and growth.

6. Acupressure

Acupressure is a technique used in TCM that involves applying gentle pressure to specific points on the body to stimulate the flow of Qi and promote healing. Incorporating acupressure into your mindfulness practice can help to support liver detoxification and enhance fertility.

There are several acupressure points that are particularly beneficial for liver health and fertility, such as Liver 3 (located on the top of the foot, between the first and second toes) and Spleen 6 (located on the inside of the lower leg, approximately four finger breadths above the ankle bone). Gently press and massage these points for a few minutes daily to stimulate liver function and support overall fertility.

7. Guided Imagery

Guided imagery is a mindfulness technique that involves using the power of the imagination to create positive mental images and feelings. This practice can be particularly helpful for women over 40 who are trying to conceive, as it can help to reduce stress, promote relaxation, and enhance fertility.

To practice guided imagery, find a quiet and comfortable space to sit or lie down. Close your eyes and take a few deep breaths to settle your body and mind. Imagine yourself in a peaceful, nurturing environment, such as a beautiful garden or a serene beach. Visualize your liver as a healthy, vibrant organ, effectively processing and eliminating toxins from your body. As you breathe, imagine this healthy energy flowing throughout your body, supporting your reproductive system and enhancing fertility. Practice this visualization for 10-15 minutes daily.

Incorporating mindfulness techniques and strategies into your daily routine can play a crucial role in supporting a fertility liver detox and enhancing overall well being for women over 40 trying to conceive.

By nurturing the mind-body connection through practices such as mindful breathing, meditation, yoga, mindful eating, emotional release techniques, acupressure, and guided imagery, you can create a supportive environment for liver health and fertility, increasing your chances of conception.

Chapter 9

Understanding Your Hormonal Profile and Fertility Tests

Introduction

In this chapter, I will explore the world of hormonal profiles and fertility tests, shedding light on the intricate connection between hormones and fertility from the perspective of Traditional Chinese Medicine (TCM).

Hormones play a vital role in our body's functions, and any imbalance can directly impact our overall health and well-being. This is particularly true for fertility, as hormones are essential for regulating the menstrual cycle, ovulation, and preparing the body for conception. TCM has a long history of addressing fertility issues by balancing the flow of Qi (energy) and nourishing the body to enhance reproductive health.

The chapter is divided into two sections, focusing on both male and female fertility. In the first section, I will explore the key tests and hormonal indicators essential for assessing male fertility and how these concepts can be applied to understand the various hormonal markers and their significance in male fertility.The second section focuses on evaluating female fertility through comprehensive testing and hormone analysis. As women in their 40s may face unique challenges in their fertility journey, understanding the role of hormones in their reproductive health becomes all the more essential. I will discuss the critical tests and hormones involved in female fertility, as well as the TCM approach to addressing any imbalances and promoting optimal reproductive health.

By gaining a comprehensive understanding of your hormonal profile and available fertility tests, you will be better equipped to navigate your fertility journey with confidence. Drawing upon the ancient wisdom of Traditional Chinese Medicine, this chapter offers valuable insights and guidance for women in their 40s who are seeking to enhance their fertility and take control of their reproducive health.

Assessing Male Fertility: Key Tests and Hormonal Indicators

From the Traditional Chinese Medicine (TCM) perspective, male fertility is influenced by a complex interplay of Qi, blood, and essence. The hormonal profile is an important aspect of this balance, especially for couples over 40 trying to conceive. As women in their 40s are researching fertility information, it's essential to understand the role of male fertility and the key tests and hormonal indicators involved.

1. Sperm Analysis: Semen Parameters and the Role of Kidney Essence

In TCM, the Kidney system plays a vital role in both male and female fertility. For men, the Kidney essence (Jing) is the foundation of reproductive function. A comprehensive sperm analysis is crucial for assessing male fertility, as it examines essential parameters such as sperm count, volume, motility, and morphology

2. Hormonal Evaluation: Key Hormones and Their Significance in TCM

A hormonal evaluation is another crucial aspect of assessing male fertility. The primary hormones involved in male reproductive health are testosterone, follicle stimulating hormone (FSH), luteinizing hormone (LH), and prolactin. In TCM, these hormones are interconnected with the balance of Yin and Yang energies and the flow of Qi in the body.

• **Testosterone:** In TCM, testosterone is closely related to the Yang energy of the Kidneys. Low testosterone levels can indicate a deficiency in Kidney Yang, which may contribute to infertility. TCM treatments aim to strengthen Kidney Yang and balance Yin-Yang energy in the body, which may improve testosterone levels and overall fertility

• **Follicle-stimulating hormone (FSH):** FSH stimulates the production of sperm in the testes. In TCM, FSH is connected to the Liver and Kidney systems. Imbalances in FSH levels may be addressed through herbal remedies and acupuncture, targeting the Liver and Kidney meridians to regulate the flow of Qi and blood.

• **Luteinizing hormone (LH):** LH triggers the production of testosterone in the testes. A deficiency in LH levels can signify an imbalance in the Liver and Kidney systems. TCM practitioners may use herbs, acupuncture, and dietary changes to support the Liver and Kidney functions, promoting the healthy production of LH.

• **Prolactin**: Elevated levels of prolactin can negatively impact fertility by inhibiting the release of FSH and LH. In TCM, excessive prolactin is often associated with a stagnation of Liver Qi. Treatment focuses on regulating Liver Qi, clearing stagnation, and balancing hormonal levels to support fertility.

3. The Importance of Holistic Assessment in TCM

In TCM, the assessment of male fertility goes beyond hormonal profiles and semen analysis. A comprehensive evaluation of the individual's overall health, lifestyle, and emotional well-being is necessary to identify imbalances and develop personalized treatment plans. TCM practitioners may also examine the tongue and pulse to gain further insight into the body's internal landscape.

In conclusion, understanding the hormonal profile and key fertility tests for men is essential for women in their 40s to research fertility information. Traditional Chinese Medicine offers a unique and holistic approach to assessing and addressing male fertility issues, taking into account the complex interplay of Qi, blood, and essence within the body. Supporting the Kidney, Liver, and overall balance of Yin and Yang energies through TCM can be beneficial for couples over 40 trying to conceive.

Evaluating Female Fertility: Comprehensive Testing and Hormone Analysis

For women over 40 who are trying to conceive, understanding the intricacies of their hormonal profile and fertility tests is essential. Traditional Chinese Medicine (TCM) takes a holistic approach to fertility by focusing on the balance of vital energy or Qi and the harmony between the various systems of the body. This sub-chapter will discuss how to evaluate female fertility from a TCM perspective, focusing on comprehensive testing and hormone analysis for women in their 40s.

Hormonal Balance and Qi

In TCM, the concept of hormonal balance is closely linked to the balance of Qi, or vital energy, which governs the proper functioning of the body. The Kidney system, in particular, is responsible for reproductive health and fertility. The harmony between the Kidney, Liver, and Spleen systems is crucial in maintaining hormonal balance and supporting conception.

As women age, their Kidney essence, or "Jing," naturally depletes, which can lead to imbalances in their hormonal profile. These imbalances may manifest as irregular menstrual cycles, changes in cervical mucus, or other fertility issues. To address these concerns, a TCM practitioner will examine the patient's overall health, lifestyle, and emotional state before recommending a personalized treatment plan.

Comprehensive Testing and Hormone Analysis

In TCM, evaluating female fertility involves examining both the physical and emotional aspects of the patient's well-being. To do this, a TCM practitioner will consider the patient's medical history, menstrual cycle patterns, and emotional health, as well as perform a thorough physical examination, including pulse and tongue diagnosis.

Alongside these assessments, a TCM practitioner may also recommend hormone tests to gain a comprehensive understanding of a woman's fertility. Some of the key hormones that play a role in fertility include:

① **Follicle-Stimulating Hormone (FSH):** FSH stimulates the growth and development of follicles in the ovaries. High FSH levels may indicate a reduced ovarian reserve, which is common in women over 40.

② **Luteinizing Hormone (LH):** LH triggers ovulation and the production of progesterone. Imbalances in LH levels can impact the regularity of ovulation, making it challenging to conceive.

③ **Estrogen:** Estrogen supports the growth and thickening of the endometrial lining, which is essential for embryo implantation. Low estrogen levels can lead to a thin endometrium, reducing the chances of successful implantation.

④ **Progesterone:** Progesterone helps to maintain the endometrial lining and is necessary for a successful pregnancy. Low progesterone levels may result in early miscarriage or difficulties in maintaining a pregnancy.

⑤ **Anti-Müllerian Hormone (AMH):** AMH is an indicator of a woman's ovarian reserve. Lower AMH levels may suggest a reduced ovarian reserve, which is common in women over 40.

Traditional Chinese Medicine Treatment Approaches

Based on the comprehensive evaluation of a woman's hormonal profile and overall health, a TCM practitioner will devise a personalized treatment plan. This plan may include:

① **Acupuncture:** Acupuncture can help regulate hormonal imbalances and improve blood flow to the reproductive organs, promoting fertility.

② **Herbal Medicine:** Herbal formulas can help nourish the Kidney system, balance hormones, and improve overall health, supporting conception and pregnancy.

③ **Diet and Lifestyle:** A TCM practitioner may recommend specific dietary and lifestyle changes to promote overall health and address any imbalances that could be impacting fertility.

④ **Stress Management:** Emotional well-being is a crucial aspect of fertility in TCM. Techniques such as meditation, Tai Chi, and Qi Gong can help reduce stress and promote emotional balance.

In conclusion, evaluating female fertility from a Traditional Chinese Medicine perspective involves a comprehensive approach that considers both the physical and emotional aspects of a woman's well-being. By examining a patient's hormonal profile and overall health, TCM practitioners can create a personalized treatment plan to address any imbalances and promote fertility.

For women in their 40s who are trying to conceive, understanding their hormonal profile and the factors that may influence their fertility is crucial.

By working closely with a TCM practitioner and undergoing comprehensive testing and hormone analysis, women can gain valuable insight into their reproductive health and identify any underlying imbalances that could be impacting their ability to conceive.

TCM treatments, such as acupuncture, herbal medicine, dietary and lifestyle changes, and stress management, can provide a holistic approach to fertility, addressing both the physical and emotional components of conception. Through these methods, TCM can help women in their 40s improve their chances of achieving a successful pregnancy and maintaining a healthy balance of body, mind, and spirit.

Chapter 10

Optimizing Fertility with Chinese Herbs and Supplements

Introduction

Traditional Chinese Medicine (TCM) has long recognized the potential of supplements and herbal remedies in optimizing fertility, offering a holistic and natural approach to promoting reproductive health.

In this chapter, "Optimizing Fertility with Chinese Herbs and Supplements," we delve into the ancient wisdom of TCM to explore the essential supplements and nutrients that can enhance fertility for both men and women, specifically for those in their 40s. Through a deeper understanding of the role these herbs and supplements play in promoting reproductive health, I aim to empower women and their partners to make informed decisions and take proactive steps in their fertility journey.

In the first section, "Boosting Male Fertility: Key Chinese Herbs and Supplements for Optimal Reproductive Health," I will investigate the vital ingredients that can strengthen sperm quality and quantity and improve overall male reproductive health. Drawing from centuries of TCM knowledge, I will identify key herbs, minerals, and nutrients that can support and invigorate male fertility.

Next, in "Enhancing Female Fertility: Key Chinese Herbs and Formulas for Optimal Reproductive Health," I will focus on the unique challenges faced by women in their 40s and discuss how

TCM-inspired supplements can nourish and balance the female reproductive system. By understanding the significance of these herbs and supplements and their impact on hormone regulation, egg quality, and overall reproductive wellness, women can harness the power of TCM to support their fertility journey.

Embarking on the path of fertility is a deeply personal and profound experience. As you explore the powerful potential of supplements through the lens of Traditional Chinese Medicine, I hope to provide guidance, insight, and reassurance, empowering you to take control of your fertility journey with confidence and optimism.

Boosting Male Fertility: Key Chinese Herbs and Supplements for Optimal Reproductive Health

In the journey towards conception, the health of both partners is crucial for successful fertilization and healthy pregnancy. This sub-chapter focuses on optimizing male fertility from a Traditional Chinese Medicine (TCM) perspective, with an emphasis on key herbs and nutrients that can improve sperm quality and quantity. This information will be particularly valuable for women over 40 trying to conceive, as they will better understand how to support their partner's fertility and overall health.

1. Traditional Chinese Medicine and Male Fertility

In TCM, fertility is influenced by the harmony and balance of Qi (life energy), Yin (female principle), Yang (male principle), and Jing (essence). Male fertility issues are often attributed to imbalances in these vital energies, which can be addressed through acupuncture, herbal medicine, and lifestyle changes, including dietary adjustments.

2. Essential Supplements and Nutrients

The following supplements and nutrients are known to promote male fertility in TCM:

a. Ginseng, Panax ginseng (Ren Shen). Ginseng is widely used in TCM for its invigorating properties and ability to strengthen Yang energy. Research has shown that ginseng can improve sperm count, motility, and testosterone levels. Regular consumption of ginseng can benefit men's overall health and fertility

b. Goji berries, Lycium barbarum (Gou Qi Zi). These nutrient-rich berries are a popular ingredient in TCM, known for their ability to nourish Yin and support Jing. Goji berries are high in antioxidants, which can protect sperm from damage and improve sperm quality. Incorporating goji berries into one's diet can have a positive impact on male fertility.

c. Maca root (Lepidium meyenii). Maca root is a popular adaptogen used to support energy levels and hormonal balance. In TCM, it is believed to nourish the Kidney Yin and Yang, which can boost male fertility. Research has shown that maca root can improve sperm production, motility, and overall sperm health.

d. Cordyceps (Cordyceps sinensis). Cordyceps is a unique fungus that has been used in TCM to strengthen the Kidney and Lung Qi. It is believed to have potent antioxidant and anti-inflammatory properties, which can support overall health and fertility. Studies have shown that Cordyceps can improve sperm count and quality, making it a valuable addition to a fertility-enhancing regimen.

e. L-carnitine. L-carnitine is an amino acid that plays a crucial role in energy production within cells. It has been shown to improve sperm motility and quality by supporting mitochondrial function. Incorporating L-carnitine into the diet can help men maintain optimal sperm health and increase their chances of successful conception.

f. Zinc. Zinc is an essential mineral that supports various bodily functions, including immune system function and cell division. In TCM, it is associated with the Kidney system, which governs reproduction. Adequate zinc intake is crucial for maintaining healthy testosterone levels and sperm production. Men should ensure they consume zinc-rich foods or consider a zinc supplement to support fertility

Enhancing Female Fertility: Key Chinese Herbs and Formulas for Optimal Reproductive Health

Traditional Chinese Medicine (TCM) has been used for thousands of years to improve fertility and support a healthy pregnancy. For women over 40 who are trying to conceive, it's essential to focus on supporting the body's overall health and vitality. Key herbs, alongside a balanced diet and lifestyle, can enhance female fertility and optimize reproductive health. In this sub-chapter, I will explore some of the most effective TCM herbs and formulas that can support women in their 40s on their journey to motherhood.

1. Dang Gui (Angelica sinensis)

Dang Gui, or Chinese Angelica root, is a powerful herb in TCM known for its ability to nourish the blood, promote blood circulation, and regulate the menstrual cycle. Women over 40 may experience irregular periods, which can make it difficult to predict ovulation and conceive. By promoting regular menstruation, Dang Gui can help improve the chances of conception. Additionally, this herb can help alleviate symptoms of menopause and improve overall hormonal balance.

2. Shu Di Huang (Rehmannia glutinosa)

Shu Di Huang, or Rehmannia, is another essential herb for nourishing the Blood and supporting the Kidney system, which is closely related to fertility in TCM. As women age, the Kidney system weakens, leading to a decline in fertility. Shu Di Huang can help to replenish the Kidney system, increase vitality, and improve overall reproductive health.

3. He Shou Wu (Polygonum multiflorum)

He Shou Wu, also known as Fo-Ti, is a popular TCM herb used to support the Liver and Kidney systems, both of which are crucial for optimal fertility. By nourishing these systems, He Shou Wu can promote hormonal balance and help regulate the menstrual cycle. Moreover, this herb is known for its antioxidant properties, which can help protect the body against age-related damage and support overall health.

4. Gou Qi Zi, Goji Berries (Lycium barbarum)

Goji berries are a nutrient-dense superfood with numerous health benefits. They are particularly rich in antioxidants, which can help protect the body from oxidative stress and support overall health. In TCM, goji berries are believed to nourish the Liver and Kidney systems, both of which play a vital role in reproductive health. Additionally, they are thought to improve the quality of eggs, increasing the chances of a successful pregnancy.

5. Maca (Lepidium meyenii)

Maca is a Peruvian plant that has been used traditionally to support fertility and hormonal balance. While not native to China, it has gained popularity in TCM due to its adaptogenic properties, which can help the body adapt to stress and maintain hormonal balance. Maca may support women over 40 by increasing energy levels, improving libido, and promoting a healthy menstrual cycle.

6. Royal Jelly

Royal jelly is a nutrient-rich substance produced by honeybees and is the exclusive food for the queen bee. It is believed to possess numerous health benefits, including boosting the immune system and supporting hormonal balance. In TCM, royal jelly is often used to improve fertility, as it is thought to nourish the Kidney and Liver systems, which are crucial for reproductive health. Additionally, royal jelly is rich in essential nutrients that can support overall vitality and well-being.

7. Zi Shen Yu Tai Pill

This herbal formula is designed to nourish the Kidney system and replenish essence, which is essential for fertility in TCM. The Kidney system weakens as women age, leading to a decline in fertility. Zi Shen Yu Tai Pill helps to support the Kidney system, restore vitality, and improve overall reproductive health. This formula often includes herbs such as Shu Di Huang (Rehmannia glutinosa), Shan Zhu Yu (Cornus officinalis), and Gou Qi Zi (Lycium barbarum).

8. Xiao Yao San (Free and Easy Wanderer)

Xiao Yao San is a classic TCM formula that aims to soothe the Liver, nourish the Blood, and harmonize the Spleen. It is particularly helpful for women who experience stress, which can negatively impact fertility. By supporting the Liver and promoting Blood circulation, Xiao Yao San can help regulate the menstrual cycle and improve the chances of conception.

9. Liu Wei Di Huang Wan (Six-Ingredient Pill with Rehmannia)

Liu Wei Di Huang Wan is another vital TCM formula that focuses on nourishing and tonifying the Yin of the Kidneys and Liver and supporting overall vitality. Composed of six key herbs, including Shu Di Huang (Rehmannia glutinosa) and Shan Yao (Dioscorea oppositifolia), this formula can help women over 40 by replenishing the Kidney and Liver system and promoting overall reproductive health.

10. Jia Wei Xiao Yao San (Augmented Free and Easy Wanderer)

Jia Wei Xiao Yao San is an enhanced version of Xiao Yao San, with additional herbs to clear heat and nourish the Blood. This formula is particularly helpful for women experiencing hormonal imbalances, irritability, or menstrual irregularities. By promoting hormonal balance and supporting the Liver, Jia Wei Xiao Yao San can improve fertility and overall well-being.

11. Gui Shao Di Huang Tang (Angelica, Peony, and Rehmannia Decoction)

This herbal formula combines the Blood-nourishing properties of Dang Gui (Angelica sinensis) and Bai Shao (White Peony Root) with the Kidney-supporting benefits of Shu Di Huang (Rehmannia glutinosa). Gui Shao Di Huang Tang is often prescribed to women with menstrual irregularities, hormonal imbalances, or Blood deficiency, which can affect fertility. By nourishing the Blood and supporting the Kidneys, this formula can help improve reproductive health and increase the chances of conception.

Traditional Chinese Medicine provides a range of supplements and herbal formulas that can be tailored to each woman's unique needs to enhance fertility and support optimal reproductive health. In addition to herbal supplementation, maintaining a balanced diet, engaging in regular exercise, and managing stress are essential for supporting overall health and well-being during the journey to motherhood.

Chapter 11

Medical Conditions and Their Impact on Fertility for Women Over 40

Many common conditions or disorders also indirectly impact fertility and you may find yourself struggling to identify and understand your own unique circumstances and how these conditions relate to infertility. Commonly encountered problems such as immune issues, infection, and advancing maternal age can all negatively impact fertility. Understanding these issues, the associated symptoms and the effects on fertility will in turn help to highlight the treatment options available and give you the best chance of a successful pregnancy in the future.

Immune-Related Factors

The immune system is an extremely complex network of organs and processes that control our body's infection response and research over the last few decades has increasingly shown that immunological factors can make a significant contribution to infertility.

Autoimmune Disease

In certain individuals, the immune system can become misdirected and begin to attack its own healthy cells and tissues in a process known as autoimmune disease. Around 20-30% of cases of recurrent miscarriage and infertility are attributed to autoimmune issues.

There are more than 80 autoimmune diseases currently known, with women being more commonly diagnosed with autoimmune diseases than men. Common autoimmune diseases include but are not limited to, Multiple Sclerosis, Diabetes, Lupus (SLE), Crohn's Disease, Antiphospholipid Syndrome (APS), allergies and Thyroid diseases, and even diseases such as Endometriosis and Polycystic Ovary Syndrome (PCOS), has been shown to include autoimmune components.

Although specific links between autoimmune disease and fertility are hard to define, there are 10 common tests that doctors can perform to identify autoimmune deficiency:

1) Anti-Sperm Antibody Test
2) Natural Killer Cell Test
3) Thyroid Peroxidase Antibody Test (TPO)
4) Anti-Phospholipid Antibody Test
5) Anti-Nuclear Antibody Test (ANA)
6) C-Reactive Protein (CRP)
7) Erythrocyte Sedimentation Rate (ESR)
8) Ferritin
9) Enzyme-Linked Immunosorbent Assay (ELISA)
10) Rheumatoid Factor (RF)

Anti-Sperm Antibody Test

Anti-sperm antibodies are unique in that they can be produced by both women and men and therefore are a commonly encountered contributor to infertility. In males, an infection or injury in the prostate or testicle can initiate the immune response. The antibodies produced can damage or destroy the spermatozoa and can in turn result in failure for the sperm to fertilize the egg.

More rarely, a woman can have a reaction to a man's sperm initiating the production of anti-sperm antibodies. Research around this phenomenon is mixed but the suggestion is that it can damage or kill sperm and as a result negatively impact fertility.

A test can be completed for anti-sperm antibodies by either taking a blood sample from a woman or a semen sample from a man. There are disputes about the reliability of this test as these antibodies can be difficult to detect but generally, there is a correlation where higher levels of antibodies found indicate a lower chance of fertilization.

The treatment for men generally involves oral steroids to suppress the immune response. For women intrauterine insemination (IUI) may help by putting the sperm directly into the uterus, as this process avoids contact with any anti-sperm antibodies which may be present in the cervical mucus.

Natural Killer Cell Test (NK)

Natural killer (NK) cells are a type of large white blood cells that play an important role in the healthy functioning of your immune system, destroying tumor cells and infectious agents among many other important tasks. However early research into natural killer cells also identified that there may be a link between the abundance of natural killer cells and failed implantation or miscarriage.

Current research into natural killer cells is mixed but there is a form of natural killer cell found in the uterus and therefore the theory is that if the placenta, embryo or fetus are mistakenly recognized as a threat, NK Cell activity may potentially lead to problems achieving or during pregnancy.

A simple blood test can indicate the number and activity levels of natural killer cells, although there is also the option to have a small biopsy taken from the uterine lining for testing.

Commonly used treatments include steroids, intralipid infusions, or intravenous gamma globulin to attempt to lower the autoimmune response.

From a Chinese medicine perspective, to lower NK cells, we employ acupuncture and Chinese herbal medicine to move Qi and Blood, nourish Yin, clear heat, and calm the Shen (nervous system). In addition, I also recommend high doses of CoQ10 and Zinc as well as an anti-inflammatory diet, reducing stress and encouraging meditation. There is a common Chinese herbal medicine formula called An Tai Yin (Calm the Fetus Decoction) which has, in my personal clinical experience, lowered NK cells.

Anti-Thyroid Antibodies (TPO)

Over 20% of women of childbearing age are positive for anti-thyroid antibodies and research has shown that women with anti-thyroid antibodies are at a greater risk of pregnancy loss and a higher risk of implantation and fertilization failure.

Hashimoto's disease is the most common form of hypothyroidism, underactive thyroid, which causes a decrease in thyroid hormone levels in the blood. With Graves' disease, your immune system attacks your thyroid gland, causing it to make more thyroid hormones than your body needs. As a result, many of your body's functions speed up. When the thyroid hormone levels are too high or too low, it can negatively affect your fertility causing difficulty with fertilization of the egg, difficulty with implantation, and increased risk for miscarriage.

A simple blood test can predict the presence of these antibodies and medication can be used to restore the thyroid hormone balance.

Anti-Phospholipid Antibodies

Anti-phospholipid antibodies result in incorrect or abnormal clotting within the blood. The antibodies mistakenly attack phospholipids—which are present in every living cell including blood cells and the lining of blood vessels. The antibodies cause damage resulting in blood clots forming in the body's veins and arteries.

When relating this situation to fertility, the presence of anti-phospholipid antibodies can prevent the correct flow of blood in the endometrium which in turn can make it difficult for implantation and in more serious cases can also cause the increased occurrence of miscarriage due to the elevation of the blood clotting mechanisms.

The most effective treatment has been shown to be anticoagulant therapy such as daily doses of aspirin or heparin, or a combination of both. Acupuncture may also assist in this situation as it has been used for thousands of years to improve blood flow.

Anti-Nuclear Antibodies (ANA)

Anti-nuclear antibodies are naturally present in our bodies to bind the contents of the cell nucleus and should be a procedure in response to foreign proteins however in some individuals the antibodies are also produced in response to normal human antigens.

With this autoimmune disorder, the whole body can be affected including impacting fertility at various stages such as affecting implantation rates and impacting oocyte quality resulting in significantly decreased pregnancy rate and increased early miscarriage rate.

Common treatment includes prednisolone (a steroid) in combination with aspirin before conception and continued into pregnancy. More natural methods to balance the immune system where high ANAs are present are to reduce stress levels and increase levels of antioxidants.

C-Reactive Protein (CRP)

The C-reactive protein (CRP) serves as an early marker of inflammation which may be associated with infertility, pregnancy loss, endometriosis, and PCOS.

Erythrocyte-Sedimentation Rate (ESR)

An erythrocyte sedimentation rate test (ESR) detects inflammation that may be caused by infection and some autoimmune diseases.

Ferritin

Ferritin is a measure of iron stores in the body and is the primary test to find out iron deficiency. High levels can indicate autoimmune disease, inflammation, infection, liver disease, or hemochromatosis. Low levels are associated with iron deficiency and we need levels above 40ng/L for optimal fertility.

Enzyme-Linked Immunosorbent Assay (ELISA)

The ELISA test is commonly used to detect antibodies in the blood. An antibody is a protein produced by the body's immune system when it detects harmful substances, called antigens.

Rheumatoid Factor (RF)

This test detects rheumatoid factor (RF) in your blood and is often used to help diagnose rheumatoid arthritis and other autoimmune disorders.

A few general tips for treating autoimmune disease naturally are:

Natural Treatment for Autoimmune Disease

• Avoid tobacco completely as it reduces basic immune defenses and raises the risk of lung and chest disease.

• Avoid alcohol and caffeine which are commonly known to impair the immune system.

• Reduce stress by practicing yoga or meditation and getting at least 8 hours of sleep a day. This will make sure levels of cortisol remain low, avoiding suppression of the immune system.

• Eat a varied diet with lots of vegetables, fruits, nuts, seeds, and those which are alkaline based or full of antioxidants. Consider taking probiotics which can reduce the risk of infection and avoid processed foods and those high in refined sugar.

• Add supplements into your diet including multivitamins, CoQ10, zinc, folate, and fish oil.

• Take the Chinese herbal remedy Zhi Bai Di Huang Wan which is used to regulate hormones naturally and can also reduce anti-sperm antibodies.

• Take herbs to support the immune system and avoid infection such as eleuthero (Ci Wu Jia), panax ginseng (Ren Shen), American ginseng (Xi Yang Shen), or astragalus (Huang Qi).

• Have several sessions of acupuncture which will improve blood flow to the uterus, regulate hormones and increase the likelihood of embryo implantation.

Over-40 Age and Fertility

As fertility challenges increasingly affect couples worldwide, many people are turning to alternative therapies to enhance their chances of conceiving. Traditional Chinese Medicine (TCM) has been practiced for thousands of years and offers a unique perspective on fertility, particularly for those over the age of 40.

This subchapter will explore the underlying principles of TCM, its approach to fertility for individuals above 40, and the potential benefits of incorporating TCM into a fertility treatment plan.

The Foundations of Traditional Chinese Medicine

TCM is rooted in the fundamental belief that the body is an interconnected system, where balance and harmony among various elements are essential for optimal health. Qi (life force energy), Yin and Yang (opposing yet complementary forces), and the Five Elements (Wood, Fire, Earth, Metal, and Water) are key concepts that guide TCM practitioners in diagnosing and treating patients.

In TCM, fertility is viewed as an expression of overall health and well-being. When there is harmony and balance in the body, fertility is more likely to be optimal. Imbalances, however, can lead to difficulties in conceiving or maintaining a pregnancy.

Addressing Fertility Challenges Over 40

As individuals age, the natural decline in fertility may be exacerbated by various factors, such as stress, poor diet, and exposure to environmental toxins. TCM offers a holistic approach to address these issues and enhance fertility for individuals over 40.

① **Acupuncture:** Acupuncture involves the insertion of thin, sterile needles into specific points on the body to stimulate Qi and improve blood flow. In the context of fertility, acupuncture can help regulate hormones, reduce stress, and improve blood flow to the reproductive organs.

② **Herbal Medicine:** TCM practitioners often prescribe customized herbal formulas to address fertility challenges. These formulas may contain herbs that enhance the quality of eggs and sperm, improve endometrial lining, and balance hormones.

③ **Diet and Lifestyle:** TCM emphasizes the importance of a balanced diet and healthy lifestyle to support fertility. Foods that nourish Yin, Yang, and Qi are recommended, as well as regular exercise and stress reduction techniques like meditation, Qi Gong or Tai Chi.

Benefits of TCM for Fertility Over 40

Integrating TCM into a fertility treatment plan offers several benefits for individuals over 40:

① **Personalized Treatment:** TCM practitioners provide customized treatments based on an individual's unique needs and circumstances, taking into account the whole person rather than just the symptoms.

② **Complementary Approach:** TCM can be used in conjunction with Western fertility treatments, such as In Vitro Fertilization (IVF) or Intrauterine Insemination (IUI), to improve success rates and overall well-being.

③ **Natural and Holistic:** TCM focuses on addressing the root causes of fertility challenges, using natural methods to restore balance and harmony within the body.

Traditional Chinese Medicine offers a unique and holistic perspective on fertility for individuals over the age of 40. By addressing the underlying imbalances in the body and promoting overall health, TCM can be an effective addition to conventional fertility treatments.

Chinese Principles of Ageing

There is an undeniable fact of life that all women must face - nature only gives each of us a small window of opportunity to have a child. This, unfortunately in most cases, starts prior to fully understanding the responsibilities of being a mother and ends significantly before we are ready to give up the opportunity of having a child!

For many women across the world, struggling to conceive as you age is not just the result of one factor but a combination of many unique issues joining together. However, age itself shouldn't be the single and only reason why you cannot have the family you desire. Looking after yourself throughout your life, by eating well and exercising regularly, can help keep your body young and significantly increase the chances of having a child later on in life.

Traditional Chinese culture perfectly exemplifies this through the principle of a woman's Qi. Leading a healthy and balanced life maintains a high level of Qi making a woman's reproductive age much lower. Maintaining this high level of Qi means that, despite your egg numbers diminishing as you get older, the quality of these eggs will not be affected and will still be released until the numbers are completely depleted.

Outside factors including stress and medication can lead to altered hormone levels which means getting pregnant as age increases becomes even more difficult. In Western medicine doctors will advise that a woman's eggs will only 'work' or be of optimal quality before a certain age or in other words, as you get ,older the quality gets worse, however, this isn't true!

In Chinese medicine, the Kidneys and Spleen are believed to be the heart of a woman's reproductive system. Keeping these organs healthy will allow the body to keep the hormones necessary for conception at their optimal level allowing pregnancy later in life to become a reality!

Natural Anti-Ageing Methods

Qi, or energy, along with blood is vital to life. In traditional Chinese medicine (TCM), the meridian system is the channel through which "Qi" or life energy moves. The female reproductive system is controlled and regulated by the HPO axis: hypothalamus, pituitary, and ovaries, which is formed when menstruation first begins in a young female.

Three important meridians; the Penetrating, Conception, and Governing meridians, align to the HPO axis. Formation of the Penetrating meridian is in the uterus making it fundamental in the Yin and Yang of the endocrine system.

Chinese philosophy states that a woman's ability to reproduce is directly related to her underlying Qi energies. The Kidneys contain this essence or vital Qi which needs to be supplemented for the duration of a woman's life through the Spleen for optimal reproductive function. Emotional well-being is also extremely important for reproduction in Chinese medicine.

Calendar age and Qi age are different but even so, a woman's essence which is known as Net Jing is said to start to decrease at the age of 49 or 50 years of age, around the time that menstruation begins to stop.

This should be a natural and slow process however environmental or physical factors including stress, illness, etc can cause Net Jing to decrease more quickly than is natural, causing a decline in a woman's fertility earlier than is necessary.

Hot flashes or mood swings are common side effects of obstructed Qi which can occur when the body is disrupted due to the sudden change in internal energy which occurs due to the transfer of energy from the uterus to the Heart as the window of fertility comes to a close.

Chinese medicine aims to regain the hormonal balance required for conception and after proper Qi-building techniques, give a woman sufficient Qi essence for all fertility requirements.

Tips to Help Achieve Pregnancy for Over 40

Any deficiencies in your body related to Qi, Kidney, and Spleen can be helped with the following tips. By creating a better Qi balance, there is no need to try and race against time for fear of missing the reproductive window!

- Get 7-8 hours of sleep each night, eat a healthy balanced diet, and adopt an exercise regime to allow your body to be in the best condition and relieve stress.

- Make an appointment with a specialist in reproductive endocrinology or a Chinese herbal medicine practitioner who specializes in fertility.

- Reduce stress by forming a network of friends, family, or external support groups who can help to support and advise you while you are trying to conceive.

- Try to be patient as healing your body will not happen overnight and therefore pregnancy is unlikely to either. It will take time so try to be patient and relaxed.

- Spend time researching alternative treatment methods that could help your unique situation.

Infectious Diseases

Not being able to conceive is arguably one of the most frustrating things for partners to experience.

Many of the tests to diagnose the issue to get pregnant will dwell on the popular failings of the reproductive system however firstly looking at simpler things, which are easier to treat, such as infection can also be extremely useful.

Prior to starting your reproductive journey, it is widely considered normal to begin antibiotics to eradicate bacteria in both the male and female reproductive systems. Using antibiotics can help with the overall health of the reproductive system increasing the chances of achieving pregnancy.

The majority of infections which can lead to infertility go unnoticed. Bacteria, for example, the resulting effects of non-symptomatic chlamydia, lead to significant scarring on the fallopian tubes, otherwise known as pelvic inflammatory disease, reducing the chance of pregnancy.

Despite popular opinion unexplained infertility due to infection in patients is not necessarily regarding sexually transmitted diseases (STDs) and their associated bacteria but can also be caused by something as common as an undiagnosed uterine infection. Other infections associated with reproductive health are:

• E-Coli
• Enterococcus
• Staphylococcus
• Ureaplasma
• Mycoplasma
• Candida Albicans (yeast)

Of course, we are not just talking about the effects that the listed infections can have on a woman's eggs and reproductive organs, they can also have a major impact on sperm. Not allowing the sperm to be able to swim effectively and reach the egg to fertilize it will obviously mean no pregnancy.

Some infections cause the sperm to stick together while others reduce the motility of the sperm so even if it reaches the egg there will not be enough energy left for it to break through the shell to achieve fertilization.

Cervical bacterial infections can also be detrimental to the sperm, so much so that even if the sperm can enter the egg it will attack the development of an embryo leading to miscarriage. It is important that if an infection is discovered in one of the partners that it is treated quickly and effectively as infections can be easily tramsmitted to each other during intercourse.

In order to improve your chances of conceiving when it comes to infections, prevention is key. Having a healthy lifestyle and eating a wide range of nutritious foods will help improve your overall immune system. Using supplements such as probiotics alongside taking antibiotics can also help to reduce the harmful bacteria while building the good!

Hormonal Imbalance

Hormonal imbalance is a common issue faced by many individuals over the age of 40. The natural aging process causes changes in the body's hormone production, leading to various physical and emotional symptoms.

Traditional Chinese Medicine (TCM) offers a unique perspective on hormonal imbalance and potential ways to address it.

Hormonal Imbalance After 40

As people age, hormone production naturally declines, leading to imbalances. In women, menopause is a significant contributor to hormonal changes, characterized by the decline of estrogen and progesterone. In men, testosterone levels decrease, leading to andropause, which presents its own set of symptoms. Common symptoms of hormonal imbalance include fatigue, weight gain, mood swings, and sleep disturbances.

Traditional Chinese Medicine and Hormonal Imbalance

TCM addresses hormonal issues by focusing on the balance of the body's energy, or Qi, and the interaction between Yin and Yang, the two complementary forces that govern the universe.

In TCM, hormonal imbalances are often attributed to the disharmony of the Kidney, Liver, and Spleen systems. The Kidney system is responsible for reproduction and aging, while the Liver system governs the smooth flow of Qi and emotions. The Spleen system is responsible for the transformation and transportation of nutrients, which are essential for hormone production.

Increased Prolactin

Prolactin is an extremely important hormone in the reproductive system as it has the potential to inhibit the production of gonadotropin-releasing hormone (GnRH) and follicle-stimulating hormone (FSH).

In turn, FSH and GnRH are the hormones that trigger ovulation and they are also involved in the maturation of eggs. For this reason, in the few months of breastfeeding, the high prolactin levels inhibit ovulation and women do not get their periods and hence do not get pregnant.

In women, high levels of prolactin in the blood can mean the hormone estrogen is not produced by the ovaries and therefore women with permanently high levels of prolactin will suffer with no period or irregular periods and struggle to get pregnant.

A simple blood test taken early in the menstrual cycle will allow an accurate evaluation of prolactin levels. Medication known as dopamine agonists (bromocriptine, cabergoline) is often used to try to regulate prolactin levels. However, there are a few simple natural methods that can help to reduce the levels of prolactin in the body:

- Concentrate on increasing your intake of certain vitamins and minerals. For example, higher levels of vitamin B6 is known to reduce prolactin as it is part of the dopamine process. Vitamin E should also be taken as it naturally inhibits the increase in prolactin levels in the body. A zinc supplement (25-40 milligrams per day) may also help lower your prolactin levels.

- Avoid nicotine and alcohol completely.

- Get 7-8 hours of sleep each night and adopt a healthy routine including meditation, yoga, and gentle exercise to reduce stress.

- Take supplements to balance hormones such as chasteberry (vitex), Qi moving herbs, and powdered ashwagandha root.

- There is also a formula in Chinese herbal medicine called Liu Wei Di Huang Wan which is used to lower prolactin (+ Rou Gui, Yin Yang Huo, and Huang Qi).

Luteal Phase Imbalance

The luteal phase occurs at the end of the menstrual cycle and several events occur during this time to encourage pregnancy. Estrogen and progesterone are produced allowing the endometrium to thicken and encouraging embryo implantation.

The luteal phase typically lasts 14 days and those that experience a shorter luteal phase have what is known as a luteal phase defect (LPD). LPD is a very common cause of pregnancy loss or infertility as the correct balance of hormones is not created within the required timeframe.

Low hormone levels such as low progesterone, FSH, and LH can cause LPD. Short menstrual cycles, irregular ovulation, multiple miscarriages, and irregular bleeding mid-cyle can all be indicative of luteal phase defects.

Testing for LPD is varied and there is unfortunately no single test that can diagnose it but there are a few common areas of investigation. Progesterone hormone levels can be tested six to eight days after ovulation as low levels may indicate a problem. Prolactin levels can also be tested as high prolactin can result in lowered progesterone.

Similarly, the investigation into thyroid hormones may be of value. TSH in particular is a clear indicator of thyroid function and can be tested simply by sending a blood sample for analysis.

Polycystic Ovary Syndrome (PCOS) is the biggest cause of infertility among women and many only find out they have it when they try to conceive. Small cysts develop on the follicles of the ovary and lead to a complex hormonal imbalance.

Higher levels of 'male hormones', androgens, are produced as a result and negatively impact the quantity and quality of eggs. Women with PCOS often have too much insulin and glucose in their blood. Diagnosis of PCOS is completed through a combination of measuring LH and FSH along with fasting glucose levels.

Modern treatments available for luteal phase defects include medications such as metformin to control glucose levels and Clomid or Letrozole to boost progesterone levels. However, these modern medications have many side effects including effects that can impact on the pregnancy itself, and therefore traditional Chinese medicine is becoming more and more popular with those looking to aid fertility in a natural way.

In the philosophy of Chinese medicine luteal phase defect is determined to be a Kidney Yang deficiency and therefore it is considered to be an imbalance impacting the whole body.

The quality of the luteal phase is a Yang deficiency and Yin and

Yang must be in balance for optimum reproductive health as Yang energy is required to create Yin energy.

This transformation of energy is created during the movement of Qi and Blood during the ovulation phase. Any imbalance of Yin or Yang at any stage in the cycle can therefore cause trapped energy and in these conditions, pregnancy will not be possible.

Herbal remedies, acupuncture, and other techniques can help to warm the Kidney Yang and nourish the Blood giving a balanced luteal phase and body temperature to aid pregnancy.

Acupuncture is used widely in the treatment of luteal phase defects. Acupuncture needles act as a tool that channel and "unblock" the disrupted flow through meridians and restore balance and thus alleviating the pain and allowing the body to heal itself.

Chasteberry (Vitex) has been shown to lengthen the luteal phase and increase the LH levels to trigger ovulation.

Red Raspberry Leaf is used in tea to increase blood flow and circulation, freeing trapped energy and increasing fertility.

Unexplained vs Secondary Infertility

Infertility is a challenging and emotionally charged issue for many couples, particularly for those over the age of 40. Infertility can be categorized into two main types: unexplained infertility and secondary infertility.

Not being able to diagnose one particular reason why you cannot conceive can be both frustrating and disheartening. Unexplained fertility can be a controversial diagnosis especially if every avenue hasn't been explored. If you are perfectly healthy and active there should be no reason why you cannot conceive right?

Unfortunately, the reproductive process is incredibly complex and relies on each component falling into place precisely at the right time. Small discrepancies such as a hormone level being lower than it should be, your womb lining being fractionally thinner than it should, or sperm not being able to penetrate the egg in time all will result in failure to conceive and often these issues go undiagnosed. However, when up-to-date medical treatment hasn't been able to provide a reason why you so far haven't been able to have a child, there are alternatives.

One of the options is to look into utilizing the treatments within traditional Chinese medicine. Traditional Chinese medicine provides a much more holistic approach to treating unexplained fertility. It doesn't focus on treating one particular aspect of reproduction which may have failed but instead looks at the bigger picture.

This may be one individual or the couple together. Initially, it is important to try and distinguish the symptoms and then focus on any trends which may be apparent. Once ascertained, a traditional Chinese medical practitioner can formulate a plan of action.

Unexplained Infertility

Unexplained infertility is a term used when doctors cannot identify the specific cause of a couple's inability to conceive. This type of infertility is more common in women over the age of 40, with an estimated 10-20% of cases remaining unexplained.

Factors such as diminished ovarian reserve, poor egg quality, and age related hormonal imbalances may contribute to unexplained infertility in older women.

Secondary Infertility

Secondary infertility occurs when a couple has successfully conceived and given birth to a child but is unable to conceive again. This type of infertility is more prevalent in women over the age of 40, as age-related factors can have a significant impact on fertility. Causes of secondary infertility may include scarring or adhesions from previous pregnancies, complications with the fallopian tubes, or changes in the male partner's sperm quality or quantity.

Risk Factors for Infertility in Women Over 40

The risk factors for both unexplained and secondary infertility in women over 40 are often similar. These can include age-related declines in fertility, lifestyle factors such as smoking, alcohol consumption, and obesity, as well as medical conditions like endometriosis, polycystic ovary syndrome (PCOS), and uterine fibroids.

The definition of infertility is the inability to have a child. When a couple mentions infertility, the initial thought is that they cannot have children at all. The situation however could be more complex in that they have been able to have one, two, or three children previously but whether it be increasing their family size or starting a new family with a different partner they are unable to do so now. This is known as secondary infertility.

Sadly, couples who already have a child generally receive less support from traditional medical routes than those who cannot have children at all. However secondary infertility comes with a great deal of emotional stress and unanswered questions.

There can be several reasons why becoming pregnant again may be difficult:

Age – Age can play a major role in the inability to get pregnant, more so if you have a hormone imbalance.

A Different Partner - If you have chosen to start a family with a new partner there could be new issues with their reproductive system that you will need to investigate.

New Health Issues - Any diagnosis or health problem which has been recently discovered should be investigated as a potential cause of infertility.

Effect of Previous Pregnancy - If there were any issues experienced during previous pregnancies which impacted your hormonal balance or physical reproductive system this could have a bearing effect on being able to get pregnant in the future.

Increased Stress - As well as having a child, life, in general, can be stressful. Having high stress levels may impact fertility and therefore changes to your lifestyle may be required in order to increase the chance of becoming pregnant.

Healing PCOS with Chinese Medicine

Polycystic Ovary Syndrome (PCOS) is a common endocrine disorder with increased androgen levels (male hormones) and/or insulin that affects women of reproductive age. As women enter their 40s, the hormonal changes that occur during this phase of life can exacerbate the symptoms of PCOS.

Traditional Chinese Medicine (TCM) has been used for thousands of years to address various health conditions, including PCOS.

Understanding PCOS

PCOS is characterized by irregular or absent periods, excessive hair growth, acne, and the presence of multiple small cysts on the ovaries. Insulin resistance, inflammation, and hormonal imbalances are common in women with PCOS. Although the exact cause is still unknown, genetic and environmental factors are believed to play a role.

TCM Perspective on PCOS

TCM views health as a balance between the body's energies: Yin, Yang, and Qi. In the case of PCOS, it is believed that an imbalance between Yin and Yang leads to stagnant Qi and Blood circulation.

This disharmony disrupts the menstrual cycle, leading to the symptoms commonly associated with PCOS. TCM practitioners aim to restore balance and harmony by addressing the root cause of the disorder, rather than just treating the symptoms.

PCOS Patterns in Chinese Medicine

In the realm of TCM, PCOS can be perceived through various lenses, often categorized as excess conditions, deficient conditions, or a blend of both. The main patterns you will see in Chinese medicine are:

1. Kidney Yang or Kidney Yin Deficiency: In TCM, the Kidneys are considered the root cause of genetic disorders and play a crucial role in PCOS. The absence of a regular menstrual cycle and ovulation is seen as a Kidney-related pathology.

2. Spleen Qi Deficiency: This pattern relates to the insulin resistance aspect of PCOS. The Spleen is responsible for the metabolism of nutrients from foods, as well as the transformation and transportation of fluids in the body. In patients with actual cysts in the ovaries, TCM considers the Spleen to be dysfunctional which creates Dampness or Phlegm. This is also the organ that relates to weight gain. Obesity is seen in 38%-88% of patients with PCOS, according to the British Medical Bulletin. By improving the function of the Spleen, TCM aims to regulate blood sugar and resolve the excess fluid accumulation from ovarian cysts and reduce weight gain.

3. Liver Qi Stagnation: Liver Qi stagnation can manifest as blood stasis or excess heat in the channels. Blood stasis in the channels can lead to excessive nourishment of hair follicles, resulting in unwanted coarse hair growth, known as hirsutism, which is a symptom often seen in PCOS patients. Excess heat in the channels also promotes the acne component of PCOS.

For both Western medicine and Chinese medicine, the first line of treatment for PCOS is nutrition, managing weight, and balancing your hormones. This involves reducing insulin levels and improving insulin sensitivity through weight loss, a low glycemic diet, and exercise to restore normal ovulation. PCOS is the biggest cause of infertility among women and from a Chinese medicine perspective, there is usually the presence of Dampness or Phlegm, which is a likely cause of PCOS.

What this means is that lots of mucus can clog up the inside of the ovaries which makes it hard for the follicles to mature and release an egg so they get stuck and many end up in there.

There is a large list of symptoms that could lead to the diagnosis of PCOS such as:

- Lethargy after eating
- Oily skin or cystic acne
- Excessive hair growth usually on the face, chin, lips and back
- Weight gain
- Irregular periods or absent periods
- Regular vaginal yeast infections
- Bright, urgent stools with a foul smell
- Painful joints
- Insulin resistance, elevated insulin levels or diabetes
- Anxiety or depression
- Cysts on the ovaries (but not always)
- Elevated DHEA and testosterone levels
- Difficulty ovulating
- Alopecia

The beauty is that PCOS responds amazingly well to changes in diet and exercise and understanding your unique diagnostic pattern will hugely impact the treatment.

Healing PCOS with Diet

A considerable amount of women who have the diagnosis of PCOS are unaware that their eating habits can also contribute to problems within their endocrine system. Simple lifestyle changes to reduce weight can improve the situation due to fat cells storing the female hormone estrogen.

It has been found that women who suffer from PCOS also have high insulin levels as the liver struggles to metabolize it. This in itself can cause symptoms as it increases the level of DHEA and testosterone in your body. In order to control your insulin levels, consider the following diet tips:

- Eliminate refined sugar, caffeine, carbohydrates, and dairy
- Eat regular meals including a wide variety of foods
- Include plenty of healthy fruits, vegetables, and salad (at least 5-9 serves daily)
- Include some protein, healthy fats, and a moderate amount of carbohydrates in every meal
- Eat unrefined carbohydrates, such as wholegrain cereals, legumes, beans, and fruit, rather than refined carbohydrates (white bread, biscuits, cakes)
- Limit saturated fats, but instead use extra virgin olive oil, avocado, nuts, and seeds, which are good sources of healthy fats
- Aim to eat more fresh foods and limit processed packaged foods
- Include prebiotics and probiotics in every meal
- Stop drinking liquid with high sugar content (fruit juice and soft drinks)
- Pay attention to portion sizes
- Increase your exercise level which means 30-40 minutes of exercise every day

Healing PCOS with Chinese Herbs

PCOS symptoms and problems associated with the condition can be treated using many herbs available. The most commonly used are:

• Gleditsia (Zao Jiao Ci) – Taking this herb regularly can help remove the waxy capsule around the ovaries that can be created by having PCOS.

• Leonurus Chinese Motherwort (Yi Mu Cao) – Promotes ovulation and blood circulation.

Healing PCOS with Acupuncture

Hormone control in the body is, as mentioned previously, controlled by the endocrine system. It has been shown that over 30% of women have found great solace in acupuncture which calms the endocrine system at the time of ovulation or reproduction. Not only this but it can regulate heart rate, breathing rate, and blood pressure as well as calm any stress.

Ovarian Cysts

Fluid-filled pockets in the ovaries are often seen in women and generally go unnoticed throughout life. Some however cause symptoms like pelvic pain and bloating. It is best that these are removed by a procedure called a laparoscopy.

Endometriosis

Endometriosis is a painful and often misunderstood medical condition that affects millions of women worldwide. Although the disease is commonly diagnosed in women during their reproductive years, it can persist and even manifest later in life. It takes an average of around 10 years to diagnose endometriosis and is also the leading cause of infertility in women today.

What is Endometriosis?

Endometriosis (endo) is a chronic condition where tissue similar to the lining of the uterus (endometrium) grows outside the uterus, forming lesions on the reproductive organs and the pelvic cavity. Endo is a whole-body disease that affects women physically and emotionally and is a chronic, progressive condition.

These growths can cause inflammation, scarring, and adhesions, leading to chronic pain and, in some cases, infertility. The severity of symptoms can vary greatly between individuals, making it difficult to diagnose and treat.

Endometriosis Over 40

While endometriosis is typically associated with younger women, it can continue to be a problem for women over 40. In some cases, the condition may even go undiagnosed until later in life. With the onset of perimenopause and menopause, hormonal fluctuations can exacerbate existing endometriosis symptoms or trigger new ones. These can include chronic pelvic pain, heavy menstrual bleeding, and dyspareunia (painful intercourse).

Additionally, women over 40 with endometriosis are at a higher risk for developing ovarian cysts and experiencing complications related to adhesions and scarring.

Although the actual cause of endometriosis is unknown, the signs and symptoms of the condition are becoming more well-known. Endometriosis is the growth of tissue usually seen in the endometrium appearing around other areas of the body, such as the fallopian tubes, ovaries, bladder, ligaments around the uterus, or the space between the uterus and the rectum. In some severe cases, it can also be seen outside the pelvic cavity such as the walls of the abdomen.

These growths can cause problems like blocking the fallopian tubes or forming scar tissue that makes it harder to get pregnant.

Some of the common symptoms include:
- Painful periods
- Heavy bleeding
- Gastrointestinal problems like IBS
- Pain during intercourse
- Bowel and bladder issues
- Ovarian cysts
- Pain during ovulation
- Hormonal imbalances
- Pelvic pain
- Severe fatigue/chronic fatigue
- Brain fog
- Depression
- Lower back pain
- Cramping
- Nausea

Tests to check for the physical clues of endometriosis include:
- Pelvic Exam
- Ultrasound
- Magnetic Resonance Imaging (MRI)
- Laparoscopy (this is the BEST way to accurately diagnose endometriosis)

Thankfully endometriosis will not stop you from getting pregnant in its mildest from however pregnancy may take more time to achieve. In more severe cases treatment can be provided to help.

The bad news when it comes to endometriosis is that there is no current cure for the condition. There are some methods that can help:

• An operation to remove the tissue in abnormal locations (excision/ablation)

• Medication to stop eggs from being released to give the areas affected time to heal

• In-vitro fertilisation (IVF)

It has been shown that the condition responds well to a diet that consists of anti-inflammatory foods, warming foods that are easier to digest, lots of cruciferous vegetables, and avoiding gluten, sugar, caffeine, red meat, and dairy. This will support the hormones, improve blood flow and reduce any inflammation.

Fibroids

Elevated hormone levels in a female's body or more specifically elevated estrogen levels can lead to fibroids. These are usually found in the endometrial walls and/or the pelvic region.

Fibroids are usually benign and are a very common occurrence ranging from the size of a marble to as large as a melon. There is no fixed number of fibroids with some women having more than others.

One major difficulty is that generally, women are oblivious to having fibroids until the struggle to get pregnant leads to investigations where they are found. It is worth noting that these fibroids, even though they can affect women of all ages, are found most commonly in ladies over the age of 35.

Uterine fibroids are non-cancerous growths in the uterus that affect a significant number of women, particularly during their reproductive years. While fibroids can occur at any age, their incidence tends to decrease after the age of 40. However, for women over 40 who still experience fibroid-related symptoms, traditional Chinese medicine (TCM) offers a holistic approach to treatment that can potentially provide relief and improve quality of life.

Understanding Fibroids Over 40

As women age, hormonal changes may lead to a decrease in the size and number of fibroids. Despite this, fibroids can still cause discomfort and complications for women over 40, such as heavy menstrual bleeding, pelvic pain, and pressure on surrounding organs. In some cases, fibroids may also contribute to fertility issues.

TCM Perspective on Fibroids

In TCM, fibroids are considered to be caused by an accumulation of stagnant Blood and Qi, often resulting from emotional stress, poor diet, and hormonal imbalances. By addressing the underlying causes, TCM aims to treat fibroids by dissolving existing growths, preventing the formation of new ones, and alleviating associated symptoms.

Fibroids are commonly treated by using systemic therapy or by having a small operation. In Chinese medicine, the alternative treatment focuses on invigorating blood circulation to promote blood flow, clear inflammation, and resolve any Liver Qi stagnation.

In some cases, fibroids will not cause a problem however, if they are affecting the anatomy of the reproductive organs and hence stopping you from getting pregnant they need to be investigated further.

General procedures, such as an ultrasound or a slightly more complex hysteroscopy will look closer at the fibroids, noting the position of the size internally. If it is deemed to be affecting your chances of implantation, then it will need to be removed.

It is becoming more common that, alongside these surgical techniques, herbal remedies and acupuncture are used to help reduce fibroids. It is very important however that if you do become pregnant while taking these remedies you should consult your local herbalist as some herbs can cause a miscarriage further down the line.

As mentioned, acupuncture can be used to help remove fibroids stimulating specific points in the uterus such as Spleen-10, Liver-4, and Bladder-17. Stimulating these points has not only been shown to remove fibroids but also stimulate blood flow.

These aren't the only methods to eliminate and prevent fibroids, other remedies include:
• Eat a healthy diet
• Reducing your body fat percentage, the more fat cells you have the more estrogen is produced
• Consume only organic meat and dairy-free substitutes
• Add artichokes and cruciferous vegetables like broccoli and cauliflower to your diet

- Reduce caffeine and sugar intake
- Avoid soy products
- Invigorate your liver by eating more radishes and adding lemon juice to water
- Consider taking supplements such as Vitamin B and omega-3 fatty acids
- Exercise regularly
- Try reducing stress in your life by taking more relaxing baths with Epsom salts

All of the above life changes can help reduce the chance of you ever having to experience fibroids. Keeping your estrogen levels normal by looking after your liver so it can remove excessive quantities of the hormone is the best place to start. This will also help blood flow around the reproductive organs. Another helpful tip not listed is to be done during menstruation itself. Placing castor oil packs in the lower abdomen region once in the morning and once in the evening can promote the workings of the lymphatic system, helping to remove the detritus from the uterus.

Fallopian Tube Blockage

To have a chance of conception, sperm is required to meet the released egg for fertilization. This most commonly occurs in the fallopian tube. If there is a blockage in either of the fallopian tubes, then it is highly likely that the chance of infertility is very high.

Fallopian tube blockage is a common cause of infertility in women, affecting around 12% of those experiencing difficulties in conceiving. Women over the age of 40 may face additional challenges in getting pregnant, as age-related factors can exacerbate the condition. Traditional Chinese Medicine (TCM) offers a holistic approach to treating fallopian tube blockage, addressing the root cause of the problem and working to improve overall health and fertility.

Causes of Fallopian Tube Blockage

Blocked fallopian tubes can be caused by various factors, including pelvic inflammatory disease, endometriosis, sexually transmitted infections, and previous surgeries. In women over 40, the likelihood of these factors contributing to fallopian tube blockage increases due to age-related changes and cumulative exposure to risk factors.

Traditional Chinese Medicine Perspective

TCM views fallopian tube blockage as a result of Qi (vital energy) and Blood stagnation in the pelvic area. This stagnation may be caused by a combination of factors, including emotional stress, poor lifestyle habits, and exposure to cold or damp environments. By addressing the underlying causes and promoting the flow of Qi and blood, TCM aims to alleviate blockage and enhance fertility.

Many women do not know that they even have blocked fallopian tubes which can be caused by chlamydia and the associated infection. Other reasons behind blockage can be down to endometriosis as previously mentioned, pelvic inflammatory disease, or adhesions from scar tissue. Regardless of the reason behind the blockage, each pathology will need its own type of treatment:

① **Thick Mucus:** Although the mucus in the fallopian tube helps direct the egg towards the womb when too much is produced it can actually create a blockage making it very difficult or even impossible for the egg to travel to where it is needed.

② **Infection and the inflammatory response:** Inflammation of the walls of the tubes caused by an infection in the entrance to the womb can make them ddhere resulting in pelvic inflammatory disease. This, in some cases, can cause long-term issues trying to conceive.

③ **Too much liquid:** Similarly to excessive amounts of mucus, infections can lead to liquid puss being created and forming a blockage. Even if the amount of puss being created isn't enough to create a blockage, it can make its way to the womb cavity affecting the development of the developing embryo.

④ **Previous scarring or thickening:** Whether it be from a previous cesarean section, distressed natural birth, or long-term infection, considerable scar tissue can stop the egg and sperm meeting for fertilization to occur

Despite the abundance of potential issues, please don't stress, in some cases, it can be fixed! Surgical removal of large amounts of mucus or fluid can be achieved by undergoing a laparoscopy. In some more severe cases, however, where there is no remedy, IVF has proven time and time again to allow you to achieve the pregnancy you desire. IVF allows the eggs to be taken directly from the ovaries, fertilized, and then re-inserted into the womb cavity to the implant, meaning the blockage in the tube will have no bearing on the results.

Successfully treating and removing blockages in the fallopian tubes differs depending on the location of the blockage. The closer to the womb cavity the blockage is, the easier it is to get a good result. In some unfortunate cases, the fallopian tubes can become blocked near to the ovary, caused by hydrosalpinx.

This forms a considerable amount of fluid which not only blocks the fallopian tube but also can be destructive to embryos if it flows into the uterus. This reduces the success rate of IVF. In this case the best advice, most likely given to you by your fertility specialist too, will be to have your fallopian tubes taken out prior to beginning IVF.

In Eastern culture and medical practices, the fallopian tubes are considered the golden pathway and must be looked after at all times, as this is what allows the egg to get to the uterus. It is understood in Chinese medicine that the narrowness and fragility of the tubes can be blocked by almost any infection stopping the journey of the egg to the welcoming warm uterus.

It is not a surprise to know that if you are wanting to get pregnant and have a child smoking will need to stop immediately. Smoking is well known to stop the small finger-like projections called cilia in the fallopian tube from directing and moving the egg toward the womb.

Although it can be more difficult, traditional Chinese medicine offers a more natural way of trying to unblock fallopian tubes. Both oral consumption and intrauterine application of herbs where they can directly pass to the tubes, promote better blood flow and reduce an inflammatory response.

Blockages caused by poor blood circulation are most frequently treated with frankincense (Ru Xiang) or myrrh (Mo Yao) in TCM. Both of these herbs are the most effective in getting to the furthest places in the fallopian tubes, especially when injected directly into the womb.

Another treatment that improves blood stasis is acupuncture. The increase in blood flow will lead to the reduction and removal of Blood and Phlegm which has become less mobile causing a blockage. Stimulating acupoints such as Spleen-10, Stomach-30, Zigong, Stomach-29, Ren-3, and Ren-4 can also help with the removal of tube blockages.

Massaging the Fallopian Tubes

Everyone is different, and some women have found that massaging the area surrounding the abdomen helps with clogged fallopian tubes. Additionally, castor oil packs can be added to the stomach area. This helps reduce significant scarring in the abdomen for example from a previous cesarean.

It is imperative that if you are considering massaging the abdomen, it is done at the right time and in the right area. The following massage for best effect should be carried out from the last day of your period until ovulation.

The locations where the massage will target are acupoints which have a link to the fallopian tubes. Starting at acupoint Stomach-

30, approximately 5 inches below the belly button and 2 inches out from the center of the abdomen make clockwise circular movements with the tips of your fingers.

Cancer

Over 1 in 2 women will develop cancer at some stage in their life but nowadays modern medicine offers amazing techniques such as chemotherapy, surgery, and radiation to help destroy the cancerous cells. The downside of many of these techniques is that they are not specific to cancer cells so generally target all cells and therefore can cause damage to ovaries, sperm, and other reproductive organs.

There are many advances in medicine that now make it possible for cancer survivors to conceive and research also shows that children of cancer survivors are NOT at a higher risk of cancer or birth defects than average. Generally speaking, women struggle more than men with infertility after cancer as the female reproductive system is much more complex with not only the initial conception of concern but the ability of the female to carry the pregnancy to full term.

Breast Cancer – Some breast cancer treatments cause temporary infertility and therefore it is generally recommended to wait a few years after having breast cancer before trying to conceive. Permanent infertility should not be an issue unless chemotherapy has permanently damaged all of the eggs in the ovaries.

Ovarian Cancer – Around 30% of patients who have multiple-agent chemotherapy suffer from ovarian failure. This situation and cases of repeated radiation or removal of the ovaries or the womb result in the need to use an egg donor or surrogate to conceive.

Uterine Cancer – The most common and effective treatment in the case of uterine cancer is the removal of the womb and in this instance, a surrogate would be required. In some cases, the ovaries and eggs may still be sufficient for use and through IVF can be fertilized and the embryo transferred to a surrogate to be carried to full term.

Cervical Cancer - Treatment for cervical cancer can increase the chance of miscarriage and also cause permanent infertility in the case of complete womb removal or long-term radiotherapy. In early-stage cancer treatment, where only part of the cervix is removed, pregnancy may still be possible but is considered to be a higher risk.

Testicular Cancer – Young men between 20-35 years old are at risk of testicular cancer with 1 in every 250 men being diagnosed in their lifetime. Treatment may include damage to the testicle or complete testicle removal and therefore it is generally recommended for men to freeze their sperm before it becomes damaged. Sperm freezes well and is stable for a long period of time so freezing should be done as soon as possible after diagnosis and before any chemotherapy or radiation treatments which can cause infertility through sperm damage or decreased sperm volume. If lymph nodes are removed or damaged, then IVF

ICSI may be required to aspirate the sperm and bypass the need for ejaculation.

As the global population continues to age, an increasing number of individuals over the age of 40 face health challenges, including cancer. Traditional Chinese Medicine (TCM) has a rich history of providing holistic and individualized treatments to address various health issues. In recent years, there has been a growing interest in the role TCM can play in cancer prevention, treatment, and management, particularly for those above 40.

The Cancer–Age Connection

Age is a significant risk factor for the development of cancer. As we age, our cells are exposed to more environmental and lifestyle factors that can lead to DNA damage and mutations, increasing the likelihood of cancerous cells forming. The risk of cancer rises significantly after the age of 40, with the majority of cancer diagnoses occurring in individuals over 65.

Traditional Chinese Medicine and Cancer Prevention

TCM emphasizes the importance of balancing the body's energy, or Qi, to promote health and prevent disease. The holistic approach of TCM takes into account an individual's physical, emotional, and spiritual well-being, which can be particularly beneficial for those over 40 looking to maintain their health. TCM practitioners may recommend lifestyle changes, herbal remedies, acupuncture, and other therapies to strengthen the immune system, reduce inflammation, and prevent cancer development.

TCM in Cancer Treatment and Management

Traditional Chinese Medicine can be an effective complementary therapy in cancer treatment, offering several potential benefits:

① **Enhancing the effects of conventional treatments:** TCM can be used alongside conventional cancer treatments such as chemotherapy and radiation, potentially improving their efficacy and reducing side effects.

② **Reducing cancer-related symptoms:** TCM therapies can help alleviate common cancer-related symptoms such as pain, fatigue, and nausea.

③ **Promoting overall well-being:** By addressing the emotional and spiritual aspects of a patient's life, TCM can improve their quality of life during and after cancer treatment.

Integrating Traditional Chinese Medicine into cancer care for individuals over 40 offers a holistic and individualized approach that can complement conventional treatments. While more research is needed to understand the full extent of TCM's benefits in cancer care, it is clear that this ancient practice has much to offer in improving the quality of life and well-being of patients.

Tubal Ligation

Tubal ligation (surgical sterilization) or the process of women getting their 'tubes tied' is a very popular procedure to prevent pregnancy but often women regret having the procedure completed and wish to reverse it at a later date.

Depending on who performed the surgery, when, and how, it may be difficult to reverse the procedure and it is also potentially damaging to fertility with the production of scar tissue, damaging infections, and an increase in the chance of ectopic pregnancy.

Tubal ligation reversal surgery should permit your eggs to travel through the tubes again by reconnecting the parts that were blocked or cut.

Recurrent Miscarriage Over 40

One of the most emotionally and physically difficult things to deal with for a couple is recurrent miscarriage. There are many causes of recurrent miscarriage including immune and hormonal disturbances. As previously mentioned, early miscarriage can be caused by incorrect levels of the progesterone hormone, and using Kidney Yang and Spleen Qi treatments can correct any abnormalities and enable the pregnancy to proceed to full term.

Recurrent miscarriage, defined as the loss of three or more consecutive pregnancies before the 20th week of gestation, can be a disheartening and challenging experience for many couples. Although miscarriages are relatively common, recurrent miscarriages can be especially difficult to navigate for women over 40, who often face additional challenges due to age-related factors.

Traditional Chinese Medicine (TCM) offers an alternative approach to managing recurrent miscarriages, focusing on holistic healing and balancing the body's energy systems.

The TCM Approach to Recurrent Miscarriage

In TCM, recurrent miscarriage is attributed to an imbalance in the body's Qi (energy), blood, and essence. These imbalances can stem from various causes, such as Kidney deficiency, Spleen deficiency, or Blood stagnation. The TCM practitioner will diagnose and treat the root cause of the miscarriage by examining the patient's overall health, lifestyle, and medical history.

Kidney Deficiency

According to TCM, the Kidneys store essence, which is vital for reproduction and growth. As women age, their Kidney essence naturally declines, which may lead to recurrent miscarriages. Treatment for Kidney deficiency often includes acupuncture, herbal remedies, and dietary modifications to strengthen the kidneys and replenish the body's essence.

Spleen Deficiency

The Spleen plays a crucial role in TCM, as it is responsible for transforming food into Qi and blood to nourish the body. A weakened Spleen may result in poor blood circulation and insufficient nourishment for the developing fetus, leading to recurrent miscarriages. To treat Spleen deficiency, TCM practitioners may recommend acupuncture, herbal formulas, and dietary adjustments to support the Spleen's function and improve blood flow.

Blood Stagnation

In TCM, Blood stagnation refers to the obstruction of blood flow, which can impede the smooth flow of Qi and cause miscarriage. This condition can be caused by various factors, such as emotional stress, trauma, or unhealthy lifestyle choices. Treatment for blood stagnation may involve acupuncture, herbal medicine, and practices such as tai chi or qigong to restore the proper circulation of Qi and blood.

Traditional Chinese Medicine offers a unique approach to addressing recurrent miscarriages in women over 40, focusing on identifying and treating the root causes of the issue rather than just the symptoms. By taking a holistic approach to treatment, TCM aims to restore balance and harmony within the body, ultimately improving the chances of a successful pregnancy.

Herbal remedies can be adopted but should be tailored to the specific issue of the individual as remedies for boosting the Blood are not applicable when miscarriages are caused by Spleen deficiency.

Some general Chinese herbs and herbal formulas to treat recurrent miscarriage are:

• Gui Pi Tang (Restore the Spleen) with herbs such as Astragalas (Huang Qi), Ginseng (Ren Shen), cooked Rehmannia Root (Shu Di Huang) can help to treat Spleen Qi issues.

• Wen Jing Tang (Warm the Menses Decoction) can be used to invigorate the Blood and dispel blood stasis where there is deficiency cold in the uterus with blood stagnation

• Asparagus Tuber (Tian Men Dong), American Ginseng (Xi Yang Shen), Ligustrum (Nu Zhen Zi), Dispacus (Xu Duan), and Cuscuta (Tu Si Zi) are the most common herbs for targeting Kidney Yin deficiency.

• Angelica Root (Dang Gui), Fleece Flower Root (He Shou Wu), and Gelatin (E Jiao) are powerful treatments for blood deficiency.

• Gui Zhi Fu Ling Wan (Cinnamon Twig and Poria Pill) can be used for blood stasis in the womb.

• Shou Tai Wan (Fetus Longevity Pill) is a brilliant formula for stabilizing any pregnancy disorders due to Kidney deficiency.

Varicoceles

The skin of the scrotum contains veins and where these become enlarged it is known as a varicocele. Varicoceles can form during puberty and they also may grow over time. They are likely to cause fertility problems in men with over 40% of men with fertility issues experiencing varicoceles. They are a common cause of low sperm quantity and quality as the temperature in the scrotum increases to higher than the ideal temperature which can damage or destroy the sperm.

Varicoceles can be easily identified due to their unique physical appearance and surgery can help to reduce them along with herbal remedies which can increase the flow of blood through the testicle.

Testicular Trauma

Testicular trauma is a wide-ranging term that includes any sort of physical damage to the testicles. Damage to testicles is common and can occur due to an accident, excessive exercise, or a physical altercation. Although TV shows may make light of the damage to the groin area in actual fact it can have severe repercussions for reproduction with surgery, medication, or treatment to reduce inflammation required to prevent any long-term impact on fertility.

Blockage of the Vas Deferens

There is a small tube within the reproductive system of the male which carries sperm and this tube is known as the vas deferens. A blockage can occur in one or both sides of the vas deferens which can result in a sperm count decrease. There are a few common causes of vas deferens blockage. Surgery in the male reproductive system of any kind can potentially cause a blockage.

The physical anatomy may be deformed from birth with congenital absence of the vas deferens possible on either only one or both sides. Where the testicle hasn't descended at puberty it can also cause a blockage and any type of infection such as chlamydia and tuberculosis are capable of blocking some or all of the vas deferens.

A more specific type of viral infection such as mumps can cause orchitis which is where there is inner and outer swelling in the testicles. In this situation the swelling can cause blockage of the vas deferens and sperm can also be killed by the virus itself.

Summary

As more individuals and couples choose to start families later in life, the prevalence of fertility challenges in the over-40 age group is on the rise. With the fertility rate dropping significantly after age 35, many couples are seeking alternative treatments to improve their chances of conceiving a child.

Traditional Chinese Medicine (TCM) has emerged as a highly effective and popular alternative, providing a renewed sense of hope and possibility for those striving to become parents.

For centuries, TCM has been utilized to treat a myriad of health issues, including infertility. A holistic and integrative approach, TCM focuses on balancing the body, mind, and spirit to optimize overall health and well-being. It includes a range of treatment modalities, such as acupuncture, herbal medicine, dietary therapy, and Qigong, which have shown immense promise in enhancing fertility in those over the age of 40.

Acupuncture, one of the most widely recognized TCM treatments, involves the insertion of thin needles into specific points on the body to stimulate energy flow, or Qi. Studies have shown that acupuncture can improve blood flow to the reproductive organs, regulate hormones, and reduce stress – factors that can significantly impact fertility. In fact, a growing body of research supports the efficacy of acupuncture in improving pregnancy rates among couples undergoing in-vitro fertilization (IVF).

Herbal medicine is another key aspect of TCM that can be tailored to the unique needs of individuals seeking to improve their fertility. By addressing hormonal imbalances, strengthening the immune system, and nourishing the body, these herbal remedies can create a more conducive environment for conception.

Dietary therapy is a further element of TCM that emphasizes the importance of consuming specific foods to promote balance and vitality. An individualized approach is taken, with a TCM practitioner recommending a diet based on the patient's unique constitution, aiming to optimize fertility and overall health.

Lastly, the practice of Qi Gong, a mind-body discipline that combines gentle movement, meditation, and focused breathing, can help reduce stress and improve energy flow in the body. Stress has been identified as a significant factor in fertility issues, and the calming effects of Qi Gong can offer both physical and mental benefits.

While age remains an important factor in fertility, the evidence supporting TCM's efficacy in enhancing fertility among individuals over 40 now has widespread acceptance.

Couples and individuals seeking an alternative to conventional fertility treatments may find solace and hope in Traditional Chinese Medicine, which offers a holistic, personalized, and natural approach to improving fertility and the chances of conception.

Chapter 12

Techniques to Boost Fertility and Reproductive Health

What Cervical Position Tells You About Your Fertility

As you embark on your journey to conceive after 40, understanding your cervical position can provide valuable insights into your fertility. The cervix, the lower part of your uterus, changes its position throughout your menstrual cycle. By monitoring these changes, you can determine the optimal time for conception. This sub-chapter will explore how to assess your cervical position and its significance in fertility for women over 40.

Why Cervical Position Matters

The position and texture of your cervix are influenced by the hormones estrogen and progesterone, which fluctuate during your menstrual cycle. These changes can help you identify your most fertile days and, in turn, improve your chances of conception. For women over 40, understanding cervical position becomes even more crucial, as the number of high-quality eggs and the frequency of ovulation may decrease with age. By tracking these changes, you can optimize your conception efforts and make the most of your fertility window.

How to Check Your Cervical Position

Before you start, ensure that your hands are clean to minimize the risk of infection. You may find it easiest to check your cervical position while in the shower or bath, as the warm water and relaxation can make the process more comfortable. Follow these steps:

① **Choose a comfortable position:** Stand with one foot elevated, squat, or sit on the toilet. Find a position that allows you to reach your cervix easily.

② **Insert your finger:** Using your index or middle finger, gently insert it into your vagina and reach upwards until you feel the cervix. It may feel similar to the tip of your nose or a slightly firmer doughnut-shaped area.

③ **Assess the position:** Notice whether your cervix feels high, medium, or low in your vagina. Keep in mind that the position may vary depending on your body and the time of day.

④ **Record your findings:** Maintain a fertility chart or use a fertility app to record your observations consistently throughout your cycle.

Understanding Cervical Position Changes

You'll notice distinct patterns throughout your menstrual cycle as you track your cervical position. These patterns provide important clues to your fertility:

① **Menstruation:** During your period, the cervix is typically low, firm, and slightly open to allow blood to flow out of the uterus.

② **After menstruation:** The cervix rises slightly and becomes firmer and closed. This phase is less fertile, as the cervix's closed position makes it harder for sperm to enter the uterus.

③ **Approaching ovulation:** As ovulation nears, the cervix moves higher, softens, and opens slightly in response to increasing estrogen levels. This is considered your most fertile time.

④ **Ovulation:** Your cervix will be at its highest, softest, and most open position, allowing sperm to pass through more easily. You may also notice increased cervical mucus during this time, which aids and protects the sperm in reaching the egg.

⑤ **After ovulation:** The cervix returns to a lower, firmer position, and the opening narrows as progesterone levels rise.

For women over 40, monitoring cervical position changes in conjunction with other fertility signs, such as basal body temperature and cervical mucus is essential. Together, these indicators can provide a comprehensive understanding of your fertility window and help maximize your chances of conception.

In conclusion, understanding and interpreting your cervical position is valuable for fertility assessment, especially for women over 40 trying to conceive. By incorporating this knowledge into your fertility journey, you can optimize your conception efforts and make the most of your unique fertility window.

Monitoring Cervical Mucus Changes

Cervical mucus plays a crucial role in conception, as it provides a favorable environment for sperm to survive and travel through the female reproductive system. Throughout your menstrual cycle, the consistency and volume of cervical mucus will change. Paying close attention to these changes can help you identify your most fertile days.

• **Dry or Sticky:** This type of cervical mucus is not conducive to sperm survival and typically indicates that you are not in your fertile window.

• **Creamy or Lotion-like**: As estrogen levels rise, your cervical mucus may become more abundant and have a creamier consistency. This phase indicates that you are approaching your fertile window but may not be there yet.

• **Watery**: Watery cervical mucus is a sign of increased fertility, as it provides a hospitable environment for sperm to swim and survive. This type of mucus often appears just before your most fertile days and indicates that ovulation is approaching.

• **Egg White**: This type of cervical mucus is considered the most fertile. It has a stretchy, egg white-like consistency, typically clear or slightly cloudy. This mucus facilitates sperm transport, nourishes the sperm, and helps it reach the egg. The presence of egg-white cervical mucus usually means that you are in your fertile window and ovulation is imminent.

Tracking Your Observations

To get the most accurate picture of your cervical position and mucus changes, it is important to consistently track your observations throughout your menstrual cycle. You can use a fertility chart, a smartphone app, or a simple notebook to record your findings. Doing so lets you identify patterns and better predict your most fertile days.

Combining Cervical Position and Mucus Observations with other Fertility Indicators

While monitoring your cervical position and mucus changes can provide valuable information about your fertility, combining these observations with other fertility indicators can help increase your chances of conception. Some additional methods include tracking your basal body temperature, using ovulation predictor kits, and monitoring changes in your cervix using fertility awareness-based methods.

Successfully evaluating your cervix and cervical position requires patience and persistence. Becoming familiar with the changes that occur throughout your menstrual cycle may take several cycles. Don't be discouraged if it takes some time to understand your body's unique patterns.

Reproductive Femoral Artery Massage

Traditional Chinese Medicine (TCM) offers a unique and holistic approach to enhancing fertility in women over 40. One such method involves the Femoral Artery Massage, which focuses on increasing blood flow to the reproductive organs, improving egg quality, and supporting overall fertility. This sub-chapter will explore the benefits of the Reproductive Femoral Artery Massage and provide detailed instructions on how to perform it.

How to Improve Egg Quality with the Femoral Artery Massage

Traditional Chinese Medicine believes that improving blood circulation and energy (Qi) flow to the reproductive organs can enhance fertility and improve egg quality. The Femoral Artery Massage works by stimulating the femoral artery, the main blood vessel that supplies the reproductive organs, legs, and lower body. By massaging this area, you can increase blood flow to the pelvic region, nourishing the ovaries and uterus and promoting healthier eggs.

Instructions on How to Massage the Femoral Artery to Improve Egg Quality

To perform the Femoral Artery Massage, follow these simple steps:

① **Find a comfortable position:** Sit or lie down in a relaxed position, ensuring that your legs are uncrossed to allow for better circulation.

② **Locate the femoral artery:** The femoral artery can be found in the groin area, where your leg meets your torso. Press gently with your fingers to feel the pulse of the artery.

③ **Apply gentle pressure:** Using your fingers or the palm of your hand, apply gentle but firm pressure on the femoral artery. Hold the pressure for 30 to 45 seconds.

④ **Release the pressure and let the blood flow normally.** When the hold is released, you should feel a sensation of warmth running down your leg as the blood supply returns to the lower extremity.

⑤ **Repeat on the opposite and perform this massage sequence** three times in a row, twice a day, from the last day of your period until ovulation, or the day before embryo transfer and not beyond.

⑥ **Do not perform this massage if** you might be pregnant or if you have high blood pressure, heart disease, circulatory problems, or a history of stroke.

It is essential to consult a TCM practitioner or your healthcare provider before starting the Femoral Artery Massage, especially if you have any pre-existing medical conditions or concerns.

Other Fertility Benefits for the Femoral Massage

In addition to improving egg quality, the Femoral Artery Massage offers several other fertility benefits:

① **Reducing stress:** Massages can help to relieve stress, a common factor that can negatively impact fertility. By relaxing the body and mind, you can create a more conducive environment for conception.

② **Balancing hormones:** By promoting better blood flow to the reproductive organs, the Femoral Artery Massage can help to balance hormones, regulate menstrual cycles, and support ovulation.

③ **Detoxification:** The massage can also aid in detoxification by stimulating the lymphatic system, helping to eliminate waste and toxins from the body.

④ **Enhancing overall health:** Improved circulation not only benefits the reproductive system but also supports overall health and well-being. Increased blood flow to the lower body can help to alleviate common issues such as leg cramps, varicose veins, and cold feet.

The Femoral Artery Massage can be a valuable addition to your fertility journey, particularly for women over 40 who are looking to improve egg quality and optimize their chances of conception. Remember to consult with a TCM practitioner or your healthcare provider before beginning any new health practices to ensure they are suitable for your individual needs.

Abdominal Gua-Sha for Fertility

Gua-Sha is an ancient traditional Chinese medicine (TCM) technique used to promote healing and overall wellness. This technique involves the use of a rounded tool to scrape the skin, stimulating blood circulation, and eliminating blockages in the body. In recent years, Gua-Sha has gained popularity for its potential benefits in supporting fertility, particularly for women over 40 trying to conceive. This sub-chapter will discuss the concept of Gua-Sha, its potential benefits for fertility, and how to perform abdominal Gua-Sha to increase blood flow to the uterus.

What is Gua-Sha?

Gua-Sha, which translates to "scraping away illness," is a therapeutic technique that has been practiced in TCM for centuries. It involves the use of a smooth-edged tool, typically made from jade, bone, or stainless steel, to gently scrape the skin's surface. This action stimulates blood circulation, breaks up stagnant energy (known as "Qi" in TCM), and releases toxins from the body.

In TCM, it is believed that energy blockages and poor circulation can lead to various health issues, including infertility. By removing these blockages and promoting healthy blood flow, Gua-Sha may help improve overall health and support the body's natural reproductive processes

How Abdominal Gua-Sha can Boost Fertility

The potential benefits of abdominal Gua-Sha for fertility lie in its ability to improve circulation and promote a healthy flow of Qi in the body. In TCM, the abdomen is considered the center of the body's energy, and a healthy flow of Qi in this area is essential for overall wellness and fertility.

When Performed on the Abdominal Area, Gua-Sha May Help

① **Increase blood flow to the uterus and pelvic organs:** Improved circulation may help nourish the uterus and create a more favorable environment for conception.

② **Regulate hormones:** By stimulating the endocrine system, Gua-Sha may help balance hormone levels, which can be particularly beneficial for women over 40 experiencing hormonal imbalances.

③ **Reduce stress and inflammation:** Gua-Sha may help relieve stress and inflammation, both of which can negatively impact fertility

④ **Improve digestion and absorption of nutrients:** A healthy digestive system is crucial for maintaining overall health and providing the necessary nutrients for a developing fetus.

Instructions on to Perform Abdominal Gua-Sha to Increase Blood Flow to the Uterus

Before beginning abdominal Gua-Sha, it is essential to consult with a qualified TCM practitioner, especially if you are trying to conceive. The following instructions are a general guideline and should be adapted to your individual needs under professional guidance.

1. **Choose a comfortable, quiet space** where you can relax and focus on the treatment.

2. **Apply a generous amount of castor oil** or massage oil to the abdominal area to reduce friction during the Gua-Sha process.

3. **Hold the Gua-Sha tool at a 30-degree angle to the skin**, with the rounded edge facing down.

4. **Starting from the pubic bone,** use gentle, even strokes to scrape the skin in an upward motion towards the naval, and then move diagonally across the ovaries and towards the hips.

5. **Work your way outwards from the center of the abdomen**, focusing on the lower abdominal area where the uterus and ovaries are located.

6. **Repeat the scraping motion for about 5-10 minutes**, being mindful not to apply too much pressure or cause discomfort.

7. **After the treatment,** take a moment to rest and allow your body to adjust to the increased circulation.

Performing abdominal Gua-Sha consistently, along with other supportive TCM practices and a healthy lifestyle, may help improve fertility and overall health for women over 40.

Castor Oil Packs for Fertility

Traditional Chinese Medicine (TCM) offers a variety of natural remedies and therapies to help support women's reproductive health. One such therapy is the use of castor oil packs, which have been utilized in TCM for centuries to promote overall wellness and fertility. This sub-chapter will discuss the nature of castor oil, how to prepare and apply castor oil packs, when and how often to use them, and precautions to take when incorporating them into your fertility journey.

What is Castor Oil?

Castor oil is a vegetable oil derived from the seeds of the castor plant (Ricinus communis). It has a thick, viscous consistency and a unique chemical composition, which gives it various therapeutic properties. In TCM, castor oil is believed to have warming and nourishing qualities, making it beneficial for balancing the body's energy (Qi) and blood circulation. These properties make castor oil a valuable natural remedy for supporting reproductive health and improving fertility in women over 40.

What is a Castor Oil Pack?

A castor oil pack is a simple, non-invasive external application of castor oil, usually applied to the abdomen. It consists of a cloth soaked in castor oil, which is placed in the skin and covered with plastic wrap, followed by a heating pad or hot water bottle for added warmth. The pack's purpose is to stimulate blood flow to the reproductive organs, promote detoxification, and encourage the flow of Qi, all of which can help improve fertility.

① **Gather materials:** To create a castor oil pack, you'll need the following items:
  - Organic, cold-pressed castor oil
  - A clean, cotton, flannel, or wool cloth (preferably unbleached)
  - Plastic wrap, plastic bag, sugarcane wrap, or beeswax wrap
  - A heating pad or hot water bottle
  - A towel or an old sheet to protect your clothing and surfaces

② **Prepare the cloth:** Fold the cloth into several layers, ensuring it is large enough to cover your lower abdomen comfortably. Saturate the cloth with castor oil, making sure it is well-soaked but not dripping.

③ **Apply the pack:** Lie down in a comfortable position, preferably on a towel or old sheet to protect your bedding or furniture. Place the oil-soaked cloth on your lower abdomen, covering the area between your pubic bone and your navel. Cover the cloth with plastic wrap or eco wrap to prevent the oil from staining your clothes or heating pad.

④ **Add heat:** Place a heating pad or hot water bottle on top of the plastic-covered cloth. The heat will help the castor oil penetrate deeper into the skin and tissues, enhancing its therapeutic effects. Adjust the heat to a comfortable level, ensuring it is warm but not too hot to avoid burns.

⑤ **Relax:** Leave the pack in place for 45-60 minutes, allowing yourself to rest and relax during this time. You may wish to meditate, practice deep breathing, or listen to calming music to enhance the overall experience.

⑥ **Clean up:** After removing the pack, cleanse your abdomen with warm water and mild soap. You can store the cloth in a sealed container and reuse it for future applications, adding more castor oil as needed. Each pack may be reused up to 25-30 times.

When and How Often to use Castor Oil Packs

Castor oil packs should be used consistently and strategically throughout your menstrual cycle to optimize fertility benefits. It is recommended to use castor oil packs 3-4 times per week, avoiding the days when you are menstruating. In TCM, it is believed that using castor oil packs during menstruation may interfere with the natural process of shedding the uterine lining.

To support the follicular phase of your cycle, which is the time from the end of menstruation to ovulation, you can use castor oil packs to promote circulation and balance hormones. During this phase, begin using the packs the last day of your period and continue until ovulation.

For women over 40, it may be helpful to use the packs more frequently, as the follicular phase can sometimes be shorter in older women.

Do not use a castor oil pack during your luteal phase when trying to conceive or if you are pregnant. It is also advisable not to use castor oil packs when you are in the stim phase of your IVF cycle. If you are estrogen priming, you can use castor oil packs but stop them once stims start.

If you are not trying to conceive you can use, you can use castor oil packs during the luteal phase (post-ovulation) every day for 15 to 20 minutes. However, if you suspect you may be pregnant, it is advisable to discontinue using castor oil packs to avoid any potential risks associated with their use during pregnancy.

In summary, using castor oil packs 3-4 times a week consistently during the follicular phase and up until ovulation can help improve fertility in women over 40. It is essential to listen to your body and adjust the frequency of use as needed, always prioritizing your comfort and well-being.

Precautions When Using Castor Oil Packs

While castor oil packs can be a valuable tool for supporting fertility, it is essential to consider some precautions to ensure their safe and effective use:

① **Pregnancy:** Discontinue the use of castor oil packs if you suspect or confirm pregnancy, as their effects on pregnant women are not well-studied, and it is best to err on the side of caution.

② **Menstruation:** Avoid using castor oil packs during menstruation, as TCM advises that they may interfere with the natural shedding of the uterine lining and there is also the potential to increase bleeding.

③ **Allergies or skin sensitivities:** If you have a history of allergies or skin sensitivities, it is essential to patch test castor oil on a small area of your skin before applying a full pack. If irritation or an allergic reaction occurs, discontinue use and consult a healthcare professional.

④ **IUDs or other medical devices:** If you have an intrauterine device (IUD) or any other medical device in your pelvic region, consult your healthcare provider before using castor oil packs to ensure their safety and compatibility with your specific situation.

⑤ **Heat precautions:** Always use caution when applying heat, making sure the temperature is comfortable and not too hot to avoid burns or discomfort. Additionally, avoid using castor oil packs with a heating pad or hot water bottle if you have a history of heat sensitivity or medical conditions that may be aggravated by heat exposure.

⑥ **Consult a TCM practitioner or healthcare professional:** If you are unsure about the suitability of castor oil packs for your unique fertility journey or have any pre-existing medical conditions, it is crucial to consult a qualified TCM practitioner or healthcare professional for personalized guidance.

Incorporating castor oil packs into your fertility routine can be an effective, natural way to support reproductive health and improve your chances of conception, particularly for women over 40. By following the guidelines for proper use and precautions, you can safely and confidently use this ancient TCM remedy to optimize your fertility journey.

Vaginal Steaming (Yoni Steam) - The Sacred Origin, The Herbs, and How to Steam

The Word Yoni and What it Means

The word Yoni is a Sanskrit term for the female genitalia, the womb, and the vagina. It signifies a "sacred place" and symbolizes the divine nature of femininity and its shared portal to life. In Traditional Chinese Medicine (TCM), the concept of Yoni is intricately connected to the overall balance and harmony of a woman's body, especially as it relates to fertility and reproductive health.

What is a Yoni Steam

A Yoni Steam, also known as vaginal steaming, is an ancient healing practice that involves the use of warm, herbal-infused steam to cleanse and revitalize the vagina, cervix, uterus, and entire reproductive system. This practice has been used for centuries in various cultures, including Traditional Chinese

Medicine, to promote fertility, regulate menstrual cycles, and maintain overall reproductive health.

Benefits of a Yoni Steam

For women over 40 trying to conceive, Yoni steams can offer numerous benefits, including:

① **Enhancing fertility:** Yoni steams can help improve blood circulation and energy flow in the reproductive organs, promoting a healthier environment for conception.

② **Regulating menstrual cycles:** By balancing hormones and supporting the uterus, Yoni steams can help regulate irregular menstrual cycles and alleviate painful periods.

③ **Detoxifying:** The herbal steam can help cleanse and detoxify the reproductive system, removing toxins and impurities that may be hindering fertility.

④ **Reducing stress:** The relaxing and soothing nature of a Yoni steam can help alleviate stress, which is often a significant factor in fertility issues.

When to Avoid a Yoni Steam

Although Yoni steams can provide numerous benefits, there are certain circumstances when they should be avoided:

- During pregnancy or if you suspect you might be pregnant.
- During menstruation.
- If you have an active vaginal infection or open sores.
- If you have an intrauterine device (IUD) in place.

Best Herbs for Yoni Steams

Traditional Chinese Medicine emphasizes the importance of using specific herbs tailored to an individual's unique needs. However, some common herbs often used in Yoni steams for women over 40 trying to conceive include:

① **Mugwort, Motherwort (Ai Ye):** Known for its warming properties, mugwort is believed to stimulate blood circulation and promote hormonal balance.

② **Red Raspberry Leaf:** A well-known uterine tonic, red raspberry leaf can help strengthen and tone the uterus in preparation for pregnancy.

③ **Chinese Angelica Root, Tangkuei, (Dang Gui):** Balances estrogen levels and regulates menstrual cycles, nourishes Blood, disperses cold, relieves cramps, treats amenorrhea and dysmenorrhea and improves fertility.

④ **Rosemary:** A powerful detoxifier, rosemary can help cleanse and purify the reproductive system.

⑤ **Lavender:** With its calming and soothing effects, lavender can help reduce stress and promote relaxation.

How to do a Yoni Steam

To perform a Yoni steam at home, follow these steps:

① **Choose your herbs:** Select the herbs that best suit your individual needs, either from the list above or with the guidance of a TCM practitioner.

② **Prepare the steam:** Boil water and add the herbs, allowing them to steep for about 10 minutes. Then, remove the mixture from heat and let it cool slightly.

③ **Prepare your space:** Find a comfortable, private area where you can sit or squat over the steaming herbs. You may use a special Yoni steam seat, a modified chair, or simply squat over a bowl.

④ **Steam:** Drape a large towel or blanket around your waist to trap the steam, ensuring it is directed towards your Yoni. Steam for 20-30 minutes, allowing the herbal-infused steam to permeate your vaginal area gently. During this time, focus on your breath and visualize the healing process taking place.

⑤ **Rest and reflect:** Once the Yoni steam is complete, take some time to rest and allow your body to absorb the benefits of the herbs. You may wish to journal or meditate to reflect on your experience and any emotions or insights that may have arisen.

⑥ **Clean up:** After your steam, ensure you dispose of the used herbs and clean the equipment used for steaming.

⑦ **Hydrate:** Be sure to drink plenty of water or herbal tea after your Yoni steam to support the detoxification process and replenish your body.

What to Expect After a Yoni Steam

After a Yoni steam, you may notice various physical and emotional changes. Some possible outcomes include:

① **Improved menstrual cycles:** You may find that your menstrual cycles become more regular, with less pain and discomfort during periods.

② **Increased energy and vitality:** Many women report a surge of energy and a general sense of well-being following a Yoni steam.

③ **Enhanced fertility:** As your reproductive system becomes more balanced and healthy, you may experience improved fertility.

④ **Emotional release:** Yoni steaming can facilitate the release of stored emotions, leading to a sense of lightness and emotional healing.

⑤ **Heightened connection:** The practice of Yoni steaming can deepen your connection to your body, your femininity, and your innate wisdom.

As with any holistic practice, individual experiences with Yoni steaming may vary. It is essential to listen to your body and work with a qualified TCM practitioner to ensure that this practice is suitable for your unique needs and circumstances, particularly if you are over 40 and trying to conceive.

Arvigo Techniques of Maya Abdominal Therapy

For women over 40 trying to conceive, a holistic approach is often recommended, which includes exploring alternative therapies that promote overall health and well-being. One such therapy is the Arvigo Techniques of Maya Abdominal Therapy (ATMAT), which has shown promise in supporting fertility and overall reproductive health.

What is the Arvigo Techniques of Maya Abdominal Therapy (ATMAT)

The Arvigo Techniques of Maya Abdominal Therapy is a non-invasive, external massage technique that focuses on the abdominal and pelvic regions. ATMAT is based on ancient Mayan healing practices and is aimed at promoting optimal reproductive health, fertility, and overall well-being. The primary goals of

ATMAT are to support proper alignment and blood flow to the reproductive organs, as well as to encourage the flow of Qi, or vital life energy, throughout the body.

History and Lineage of the Arvigo Techniques of Maya Abdominal Therapy

ATMAT has its roots in the Mayan culture of Central America, where traditional healers have been using these techniques for centuries to support reproductive health, fertility, and overall well-being. Dr Rosita Arvigo, a naprapathic physician and herbalist, learned these techniques from her mentor, the late Don Elijio Panti, a highly respected Mayan healer. Dr Arvigo spent many years studying and practicing with Don Elijio, refining the techniques and adapting them for use in modern clinical settings.

Today, the Arvigo Techniques of Maya Abdominal Therapy have been taught to thousands of practitioners worldwide, offering hope and support for women and men seeking to improve their reproductive health and fertility.

How Does Maya Abdominal Therapy Support Fertility

From a TCM perspective, ATMAT supports fertility by promoting proper alignment and blood flow to the reproductive organs, as well as encouraging the flow of Qi throughout the body. By gently massaging and repositioning the uterus and other reproductive organs, ATMAT helps to release physical and emotional blockages that may be impeding fertility. This can lead to improved menstrual cycles, decreased pain and discomfort associated with menstruation, and increased chances of conception.

Benefits of the Arvigo Techniques of Maya Abdominal Therapy for Men

Although this sub-chapter focuses on women over 40 trying to conceive, it is important to note that ATMAT is not exclusively beneficial for women. Men can also benefit from these techniques, as they help to promote proper blood flow and alignment of the male reproductive organs. This can lead to improved sperm production and quality, enhanced libido, and overall increased vitality.

What to Expect During Your Initial Session

During your initial session, your practitioner will gather information about your medical history, fertility journey, and any specific concerns you may have. This information will be used to tailor the treatment to your individual needs. The actual therapy will begin with a gentle, external abdominal massage, focusing on the lower abdomen and pelvic area. Your practitioner may also incorporate other elements of TCM, such as herbal medicine, acupuncture, or moxibustion, to further support your fertility journey.

The Arvigo Techniques of Maya Abdominal Therapy can be an invaluable addition to your fertility journey, particularly if you are a woman over 40 seeking to conceive. By embracing this holistic, non-invasive approach, you are supporting your body's natural ability to achieve balance and optimal reproductive health. As with any treatment, it is important to consult with a qualified practitioner and to openly discuss your individual needs and concerns.

Chapter 13

A Guide to the Best Fertility Supplements and Vitamins

Introduction

In the vast ocean of knowledge that Traditional Chinese Medicine (TCM) offers, the realm of fertility holds a special place. With time-tested wisdom and centuries of empirical evidence, TCM provides a holistic approach to enhancing fertility, particularly for women in their 40s who are seeking to conceive. Welcome to this enriching journey, as we delve into "A Guide to the Best Fertility Supplements and Vitamins" from the perspective of Traditional Chinese Medicine.

As a woman in her 40s, you may face unique challenges in your pursuit of fertility. Modern lifestyles, environmental factors, and the natural aging process can all impact your reproductive health. However, Traditional Chinese Medicine offers hope and guidance, helping you to restore balance and enhance your fertility through the use of natural supplements and vitamins. This ancient wisdom focuses on nourishing the body, mind, and spirit, ensuring that you are in the best possible state for conception.

We will explore a variety of fertility supplements and vitamins that have been proven to support and improve reproductive health in accordance with the principles of Traditional Chinese Medicine. I will delve into each supplement and vitamin's properties, providing a solid understanding of their role in promoting fertility. Additionally, I will provide recommendations on how to incorporate these supplements and vitamins into your daily routine, while paying close attention to your individual needs and constitution.

Embark on this enlightening journey as we uncover the secrets of Traditional Chinese Medicine for enhanced fertility. With patience, dedication, and a deeper understanding of the wisdom that TCM has to offer, you may find the support you need to fulfill your dreams of motherhood. May this guide serve as a beacon of hope and inspiration as you explore the natural and holistic path to fertility, guided by the ancient wisdom of Traditional Chinese Medicine.

Optimal Vitamins to Boost Female Fertility: A Comprehensive Guide

As a woman in her 40s trying to conceive, it's crucial to pay attention to the nutrients that can support your fertility journey. Traditional Chinese Medicine (TCM) considers the balance of Qi, Yin, and Yang in the body as a crucial factor for optimal health and fertility. While TCM relies primarily on herbal treatments, acupuncture, and lifestyle adjustments, incorporating the right vitamins and minerals can complement these practices and improve your fertility potential.

This comprehensive guide will outline the key vitamins and minerals to include in your diet from a TCM perspective, specifically for women over 40 trying to conceive.

Vitamin A

Vitamin A is essential for overall reproductive health, as it plays a vital role in maintaining the health of the fallopian tubes, uterus, and ovaries. In TCM, Vitamin A is believed to nourish the Yin and contribute to the overall balance of the body. The antioxidant properties of Vitamin A also help combat free radicals, which can damage cells and contribute to aging.

For women over 40, it's important to consume Vitamin A in the form of beta-carotene, found in plant-based sources like carrots, sweet potatoes, spinach, and apricots. Beta-carotene is converted into Vitamin A in the body, allowing for a safer and more controlled intake.

Vitamin E

Vitamin E is a powerful antioxidant that protects cells from oxidative stress, which can lead to DNA damage and hinder fertility. In TCM, Vitamin E is believed to nourish the Yin and blood, promoting better circulation and enhancing the overall reproductive function.

Sources of Vitamin E include nuts and seeds (like almonds, sunflower seeds, and hazelnuts), as well as leafy greens, avocado, and wheat germ oil. It's essential to incorporate these foods into your diet to support healthy egg quality and overall reproductive health.

Zinc

Zinc is a critical mineral for fertility, as it plays a role in hormone regulation, ovulation, and cell division. In TCM, Zinc is thought to promote Yang energy, nourish the Kidney Qi, and enhance fertility by balancing hormone levels and supporting the immune system.

Women over 40 should focus on consuming foods rich in zinc, such as oysters, beef, pumpkin seeds, and lentils. In some cases, zinc supplementation may be recommended to ensure optimal levels, but it's crucial to consult with a TCM practitioner or healthcare professional before starting any supplement regimen.

Folate

Folate, also known as folate or Vitamin B9, is essential for DNA synthesis and cell division, directly impacting the quality and health of eggs. In TCM, folate is considered a vital nutrient to nourish the blood and support the Spleen Qi, which is responsible for transforming and transporting nutrients throughout the body.

It's crucial for women over 40 to consume adequate amounts of folate, as deficiency can increase the risk of birth defects. Good sources of folate include leafy greens, beans, and fortified grains. Supplementation of 400 mcg of folate is recommended for women trying to conceive.

B Vitamins

The B-vitamin complex is a group of eight essential nutrients that play a critical role in overall health and fertility. B vitamins, particularly B6 and B12, are crucial for hormone regulation, ovulation, and the formation of red blood cells. In TCM, B vitamins are thought to support the Liver Qi, which is responsible for the smooth flow of Qi and blood throughout the body.

To ensure an adequate intake of B vitamins, incorporate a variety of whole grains,legumes, and lean meats into your diet. In some cases, supplementation may be necessary, especially for women following vegetarian or vegan diets, as some B vitamins, like B12, are predominantly found in animal products. In TCM, it's important to consume foods that are considered warming or neutral in nature, such as brown rice, oats, lentils, and chicken, to support the overall balance of Qi and nourish the Liver Qi.

Selenium

Selenium is a trace mineral that plays a critical role in maintaining healthy thyroid function and protecting cells from oxidative stress. In TCM, selenium is believed to nourish the Kidney Qi and support the Yin and Yang balance, which can contribute to improved fertility outcomes.

For women over 40 trying to conceive, incorporating selenium-rich foods into the diet is essential. Good sources of selenium include Brazil nuts, tuna, shrimp, and whole grains. It's important to note that selenium can be toxic in excessive amounts, so it's crucial to consult with a healthcare professional before considering supplementation.

The optimal vitamins and minerals to support fertility in women over 40 from a TCM perspective include Vitamin A, Vitamin E, Zinc, Folate, B vitamins, and Selenium. By incorporating these nutrients into your diet and working closely with a TCM practitioner or healthcare professional, you can create a balanced and nourishing environment to support your fertility journey. Remember that lifestyle factors, such as stress management, exercise, and sleep, also play a crucial role in ferility, so be sure to address these aspects in addition to your nutritional needs.

Top Supplements to Enhance Female Fertility: What You Need to Know

As women reach their 40s, the journey to conceive can become more challenging due to age-related factors. However, Traditional Chinese Medicine (TCM) offers various time-tested approaches to support and enhance female fertility.

One such approach involves incorporating specific supplements and vitamins into your daily routine. In this sub-chapter, we will explore the best fertility supplements and vitamins from a TCM perspective for women over 40 trying to conceive.

Preconception Multivitamin for Women

A preconception multivitamin is a specially formulated supplement designed to support women's health before and during pregnancy. These vitamins typically contain a blend of essential nutrients, such as folate, iron, and iodine, which are crucial for the development of a healthy baby. From a TCM standpoint, a balanced preconception vitamin can help nourish the body, maintain overall health, and improve the chances of conception.

Coenzyme Q10 (CoQ10)

Coenzyme Q10, or CoQ10, is a powerful antioxidant that plays a crucial role in energy production within cells. In TCM, CoQ10 is believed to support the Kidney system, which governs fertility and reproductive health. As women age, their natural levels of CoQ10 decrease, which can negatively impact egg quality and energy levels. Supplementing with CoQ10 can help improve egg quality, maintain optimal energy levels, and promote overall reproductive health.

Omega-3 Fatty Acids

Omega-3 fatty acids are essential nutrients known for their anti-inflammatory and cardiovascular benefits. In TCM, omega-3s are considered vital for nourishing the liver and Kidney systems, both of which play significant roles in fertility. For women over 40 trying to conceive, incorporating omega-3 fatty acids into their diet or through supplementation can help reduce inflammation, support hormonal balance, and improve the quality of the uterine environment.

Magnesium

Magnesium is an essential mineral that plays a critical role in over 300 biochemical reactions in the body, including those related to the reproductive system. In TCM, magnesium is known to support the Spleen and Kidney systems, both of which are involved in fertility. For women over 40, magnesium supplementation can help maintain hormonal balance, reduce stress levels, and support a healthy uterine lining, thus improving the chances of conception.

Probiotics

Probiotics are beneficial bacteria that help maintain a healthy gut microbiome, which plays a crucial role in overall health, including reproductive health. In TCM, the gut is considered the foundation of health, and a healthy gut is vital for optimal fertility. As women age, their gut microbiome can change, leading to imbalances that may affect their ability to conceive. By incorporating probiotics into their daily routine, women over 40 can support a healthy gut environment, improve digestion and absorption of nutrients, and promote hormonal balance, all of which can enhance fertility.

The journey to conception can be challenging for women over 40, but incorporating these supplements and vitamins into your daily routine can significantly enhance your fertility. By nourishing the body and supporting the key organ systems involved in reproductive health from a TCM perspective, you can improve your chances of achieving a healthy pregnancy. Always consult with a healthcare professional or TCM practitioner before starting any new supplement regimen to ensure it is safe and appropriate for your individual needs.

Essential Vitamins for Male Fertility: A Complete Overview

This sub-chapter focuses on essential vitamins and minerals that contribute to male fertility, which can also be beneficial for women in their 40s who are researching fertility information for themselves.

Zinc

Zinc is an essential trace element that plays a crucial role in male fertility. In TCM, zinc is known to strengthen the Kidney Qi, which is essential for maintaining reproductive health. A deficiency in zinc can lead to poor sperm quality, low sperm count, and impaired sperm motility. It is important for men to consume adequate amounts of zinc through their diet or by taking supplements. Foods rich in zinc include oysters, red meat, poultry, beans, nuts, and whole grains.

Folate

Folate, also known as Vitamin B9, is important for both male and female fertility. In men, folate is required for the synthesis of DNA and RNA, which is essential for sperm production and function. A deficiency in folate can lead to abnormal sperm, reduced sperm count, and an increased risk of chromosomal abnormalities. Foods rich in folate include dark leafy greens, beans, lentils, and fortified cereals.

Vitamin C

Vitamin C is a powerful antioxidant that plays an essential role in protecting sperm from oxidative stress and damage. In TCM, Vitamin C is believed to support the liver Qi, which is responsible for the smooth flow of Qi and blood throughout the body. This helps to maintain a healthy reproductive system in both men and women. Men should consume adequate amounts of Vitamin C through their diet or by taking supplements. Foods rich in Vitamin C include citrus fruits, berries, kiwi, melons, and peppers.

Selenium

Selenium is an essential trace element that plays a vital role in male fertility by supporting sperm formation and function. In TCM, selenium is believed to nourish the Kidney Essence and promote overall vitality, which is essential for reproductive health. A deficiency in selenium can lead to poor sperm quality and reduced fertility. Foods rich in selenium include Brazil nuts, tuna, beef, chicken, and eggs.

Vitamin E

Vitamin E is a powerful antioxidant that helps protect sperm from oxidative stress and damage. In TCM, Vitamin E is believed to support the Liver Qi and nourish the Kidney Essence, contributing to healthy blood circulation and overall vitality. Adequate Vitamin E intake can improve sperm quality, motility, and overall fertility. Foods rich in Vitamin E include almonds, sunflower seeds, avocados, spinach, and vegetable oils.

Vitamin D

Vitamin D is essential for maintaining overall health and well-being, including reproductive health. In TCM, Vitamin D is believed to nourish the Kidney Essence, which is essential for maintaining reproductive health. Low levels of Vitamin D have been associated with poor sperm quality, reduced sperm count, and impaired sperm motility. Men should ensure they receive adequate amounts of Vitamin D through sun exposure, diet, or supplements. Foods rich in Vitamin D include fatty fish, egg yolks, and salmon.

Maintaining a healthy balance of essential vitamins and minerals is vital for male fertility, which can have a significant impact on the chances of conception for women.

The Ultimate Guide to Supplements for Boosting Male Fertility

Preconception Multivitamin for Men

Preconception multivitamins are designed to help provide essential nutrients to men in preparation for conception. In TCM, the concept of "Jing" is vital to fertility. Jing is the essence of life and is believed to be responsible for reproductive health, among other things. When the Jing is strong and well-nourished, fertility is enhanced.

A high-quality preconception multivitamin for men should contain a blend of vitamins, minerals, and antioxidants that support sperm health and overall male reproductive function. Key ingredients may include zinc, selenium, vitamin C, and vitamin E. These nutrients work together to nourish Jing and boost fertility from a TCM standpoint.

Coenzyme Q10 (CoQ10)

Coenzyme Q10, also known as CoQ10, is a powerful antioxidant that plays a crucial role in cellular energy production. In TCM, it is believed that healthy sperm requires an abundance of energy, or Qi, to function optimally. CoQ10 can help increase this energy, leading to improved sperm motility and overall male fertility.

Research has shown that CoQ10 supplementation can significantly improve sperm parameters, including concentration, motility, and morphology. For men over 40, CoQ10 supplementation becomes even more critical, as natural CoQ10 levels decline with age. A daily dose of 600 mg of CoQ10 is typically recommended to support fertility.

Omega-3 Fatty Acids

Omega-3 fatty acids are essential nutrients that are crucial to overall health and fertility. From a TCM perspective, omega-3s help to nourish the Kidney system, which is responsible for storing Jing and maintaining reproductive health. By supporting the Kidney system, omega-3 fatty acids can contribute to improved sperm quality and overall male fertility.

Foods rich in omega-3 fatty acids include fish, nuts, and seeds.

However, a supplement containing EPA and DHA is recommended for those who do not consume enough omega-3s in their diet. A daily dose of 2000-4000 mg of combined EPA and DHA can provide essential support for male fertility.

L-Carntine

L-Carnitine is an amino acid that plays a vital role in cellular energy production, specifically in the transport of fatty acids into the mitochondria to be used as fuel.

In TCM, sperm requires abundant Qi to function optimally, and L-Carnitine's role in energy production aligns with this belief.

Studies have demonstrated that L-Carnitine supplementation can improve sperm motility, concentration, and overall fertility. For men over 40, supplementing with L-Carnitine can be particularly beneficial due to age-related declines in sperm quality. A daily dose of 1000-3000 mg of L-Carnitine is typically recommended to support male fertility.

Probiotics

Probiotics are beneficial microorganisms that promote a healthy balance of gut bacteria. Maintaining a healthy gut environment is crucial for overall health and wellbeing. A healthy gut can improve nutrient absorption, support immune function, and regulate inflammation – all factors that can impact fertility.

As men age, the balance of gut bacteria can become disrupted, which may contribute to a variety of health issues, including those that impact fertility. In TCM, maintaining a healthy gut is believed to support the Spleen and Stomach systems, which are responsible for transforming and transporting nutrients throughout the body. By nourishing these systems, overall health and fertility can be improved.

Probiotic supplements can help restore and maintain a healthy balance of gut bacteria, supporting digestion, nutrient absorption, and immune function. For men over 40, taking a daily probiotic supplement containing a variety of beneficial strains, such as Lactobacillus and Bifidobacterium, can be beneficial in promoting gut health and supporting fertility.

In conclusion, Traditional Chinese Medicine offers valuable insights into the importance of nourishing the body and optimizing fertility, particularly for couples in their 40s trying to conceive. By incorporating a preconception multivitamin, CoQ10, omega-3 fatty acids, L-Carnitine, and probiotics into your daily routine, you can support your partner's reproductive health and enhance your chances of successful conception. It is essential to consult with a qualified healthcare practitioner or TCM practitioner to discuss your individual needs and determine the most appropriate supplements and dosages for your unique situation.

Additional Antioxidants Worth Considering for Improved Health

For women over 40, fertility can be more challenging due to the natural decline in ovarian function and egg quality. This sub-chapter will discuss additional antioxidants and supplements that can be beneficial for women in their 40s trying to conceive. These antioxidants can help improve overall health and promote amore balanced internal environment, increasing the chances of successful conception.

Alpha-Lipoic Acid

Alpha-lipoic acid is a potent antioxidant that assists in combating oxidative stress, which can have negative effects on fertility. By reducing inflammation and supporting cellular energy production, alpha-lipoic acid can help improve egg quality in women over 40. In TCM, this supplement aids in promoting a balance between Yin and Yang and may improve overall reproductive health.

N-Acetyl Cysteine

N-acetyl cysteine (NAC) is a powerful antioxidant that can support fertility by reducing oxidative stress and inflammation. NAC can help protect egg quality, which is essential for women over 40 who may experience a decline in egg health due to age. In TCM, NAC is believed to nourish the Kidney Yin, which is associated with reproductive vitality.

Melatonin

Melatonin is a hormone that regulates sleep and is also a powerful antioxidant. Studies have shown that melatonin can protect eggs from oxidative stress, improving their quality and increasing the chances of successful conception. Melatonin supplementation can also support the natural circadian rhythm, which is essential for hormonal balance in TCM.

Myo-Inositol for Women with PCOS to Improve Ovulation and Who have Insulin Resistance

Myo-inositol is a vitamin-like substance that has been shown to help women with polycystic ovary syndrome (PCOS) and insulin resistance by improving ovulation and regulating blood sugar levels. In TCM, myo-inositol can help regulate Qi and support the Spleen, which is associated with proper digestion and blood sugar balance.

Glutathione

Glutathione is a powerful antioxidant that supports detoxification and protects cells from oxidative damage. For women over 40, glutathione can help improve egg quality and support overall reproductive health. In TCM, glutathione can help strengthen the Liver, which is responsible for detoxification and blood circulation.

Maca

Maca is a Peruvian plant that has been used for centuries to enhance fertility and libido. It is rich in antioxidants and can help support hormonal balance in women over 40, thereby promoting healthy reproductive function. Maca can be considered an adaptogen in TCM, helping the body adapt to stress and maintain a healthy balance between Yin and Yang.

Resveratol

Resveratrol is a powerful antioxidant found in the skin of red grapes, which has been shown to improve ovarian function and support healthy aging. In women over 40, resveratrol can help improve egg quality and overall reproductive health. In TCM, resveratrol is believed to support the Blood and Qi, promoting proper circulation and nourishment of the reproductive organs.

DHEA

Dehydroepiandrosterone (DHEA) is a hormone that naturally declines with age. Studies have shown that DHEA supplementation can improve egg quality in women over 40, increasing the chances of successful conception. In TCM, DHEA supports the Kidney Yang, which is associated with reproductive warmth and vitality.

Chapter 14

Tantra: The Art of Sexual Ecstasy

Introduction

In this enlightening chapter, I delve into the world of Tantra, an ancient practice that transcends the physical realm, connecting the mind, body, and spirit to enhance fertility and sexual pleasure. Emphasizing the principles of Traditional Chinese Medicine, I cater specifically to women in their 40s, seeking to empower them on their journey to better understand their bodies, increase intimacy with their partners, and awaken their full potential for fertility.

As I explore the history of Tantra, I will unveil the rich tapestry of its origins and the profound impact it has had on countless lives over the millennia. Through understanding the four essentials of Tantra sex teachings, you will discover the power of conscious creation and how to prepare yourself to host a soul.

Contrary to popular belief, Tantra is not solely about sex. Instead, it is an intricate study of energy and spiritual sexuality. I will guide you through the steps to harness your innate sexual energy and channel it into the art of lovemaking, fostering deeper connections and enhancing fertility.

Strengthening the bond between you and your partner is central to Tantra. I will discuss the many ways Tantra can cultivate love and intimacy in relationships, ultimately creating an ideal environment for conception. I will also delve into the fascinating world of the seven different types of female orgasms, offering insight into the unique experiences of pleasure and their significance in fertility.

For men, I will clarify the distinction between orgasm and ejaculation and introduce semen retention, a powerful practice that allows for greater control over one's sexual energy. By mastering these techniques, couples can enhance their lovemaking and significantly increase their chances of conception.

Finally, I will provide a comprehensive guide to various Tantra sexual practices designed to facilitate conscious conception. These transformative techniques, including soul gazing, Tantric and Taoist massage and bodywork, genital mapping, and womb meditation, will not only create a deeper connection with yourself and your partner but also foster a sacred space for new life to flourish.

I encourage you to embrace this journey of self-discovery and spiritual awakening, the wisdom of Tantra, and its incredible potential to transform your fertility, relationships, and overall well-being.

The History of Tantra

The ancient art of Tantra has been practiced for thousands of years, with its roots traced back to India, China, and Tibet. Tantra, a Sanskrit word that can be translated to "lave" or "loom," is an esoteric spiritual practice that aims to have together the physical, emotional, and spiritual aspects of life. As a holistic approach to well-being, Tantra has been incorporated into Traditional Chinese Medicine (TCM) to address various aspects of health, including fertility.

Origins and Development of Tantra

While Tantra's origins are believed to date back to prehistoric India, its influence spread across Asia over the centuries, eventually making its way to China, where it blended with existing philosophies and practices. The incorporation of Tantra into Chinese culture took place around the 8th century CE, during the Tang Dynasty when Chinese Buddhists began adopting Tantric practices into their spiritual routines.

As Tantra was assimilated into Chinese culture, it became increasingly intertwined with Traditional Chinese Medicine (TCM). The TCM perspective on fertility is holistic, emphasizing the importance of balance and harmony within the body. This is achieved by considering the flow of Qi (life energy), the balance of Yin and Yang, and the health of the meridians that channel energy throughout the body.

Tantra's emphasis on spiritual and physical balance complemented TCM's approach to fertility, making it a natural addition to the Chinese medicinal system.

The Role of Tantra in Fertility

For women over 40 who are trying to conceive, incorporating Tantric practices into their fertility journey can provide a holistic approach that addresses both the physical and emotional aspects of fertility. From a TCM perspective, Tantra can help women:

① **Balance the Yin and Yang:** Achieving a harmonious balance between Yin (the feminine, nurturing energy) and Yang (the masculine, active energy) is crucial for optimal fertility. Tantric practices, such as specific meditation techniques, yoga poses, and breathing exercises, can help to restore this balance and promote a healthy environment for conception.

② **Strengthen the Qi and Blood:** According to TCM, the flow of Qi and the quality of Blood are both essential for reproductive health. Tantra's emphasis on physical health through diet, exercise, and relaxation can support the body in maintaining strong Qi and nourishing Blood, which can enhance fertility.

③ **Cultivate Emotional Well-Being:** Emotional health is often overlooked when addressing fertility issues, but it plays a crucial role in conception. Tantric practices can help women connect with their emotions, release negative energy, and build resilience, which can support their journey toward motherhood.

④ **Enhance Sexual Energy:** Tantra places a strong focus on sexual energy as a source of vitality and life force. For women over 40 trying to conceive, tapping into this energy through Tantric practices can help to increase sexual desire, improve sexual function, and promote a deeper connection with their partners, all of which can contribute to improved fertility outcomes.

Applying Tantra to your Fertility Journey

To incorporate Tantric practices into your fertility journey, consider working with a qualified TCM practitioner who is knowledgeable about Tantra. They can guide you through the various techniques and provide personalized advice based on your specific needs and goals. It is essential to approach Tantra with an open mind and a willingness to explore the various physical, emotional, and spiritual aspects of the practice.

Tantra has a rich history as a spiritual practice that has been incorporated into Traditional Chinese Medicine to address various health concerns, including fertility.

For women over 40 trying to conceive, embracing Tantra's holistic approach to health and well-being can help to restore balance, enhance vitality, and support emotional resilience, all of which can contribute to improved fertility.

What is Tantra?

The art of Tantra has captivated the interest of many individuals across the globe, with its sensual and mystical approach to sexuality, relationships, and spirituality. However, it is essential to understand that Tantra is not solely about sex, but rather about a deeper connection with yourself and your partner.

This sub-chapter, written from a Traditional Chinese Medicine perspective, will discuss the practice of Tantra and its potential benefits for women over 40 trying to conceive.

Origins and Philosophy of Tantra

Tantra has its roots in ancient Indian spiritual traditions, dating back to over 5,000 years ago. The word "tantra" is derived from two Sanskrit words: "tanoti," which means "to expand," and "trayati," meaning "to liberate." In essence, Tantra is a practice that aims to expand one's consciousness and liberate oneself from the confines of ego and societal expectations, allowing for a deeper understanding of the self and the world.

From a Traditional Chinese Medicine (TCM) perspective, Tantra shares similarities with the Taoist practices of cultivating life force energy (Qi) and balancing the energies of Yin and Yang. By integrating the principles of TCM and Tantra, women over 40 can potentially enhance their fertility by balancing their energies, reducing stress, and nurturing their body, mind, and spirit.

Tantra and Sexual Energy

In the practice of Tantra, sexual energy is regarded as a powerful life force that can be harnessed for personal growth, self-awareness, and healing. Tantra teaches that the union of male and female energies (symbolized by the Yin and Yang in TCM) can lead to spiritual and physical harmony, which may, in turn, have a positive impact on fertility.

For women over 40, engaging in Tantra can help to balance hormonal levels, improve blood circulation, and reduce stress – all of which are essential factors for successful conception. Moreover, the practice of Tantra emphasizes the importance of emotional intimacy, creating a deeper bond between partners that can lead to a more nurturing and supportive environment for conception.

Practical Techniques for Enchancing Fertility

Here are some practical Tantra techniques that women over 40 can incorporate into their daily lives to boost fertility:

① **Meditation and Visualization:** Engaging in regular meditation and visualization practices can help calm the mind, balance hormones, and improve the flow of Qi in the body. Focus on visualizing your womb as a nurturing, vibrant, and healthy space for new life.

② **Breathwork:** Practicing deep, slow, and mindful breathing can reduce stress, improve oxygen levels, and enhance overall Ill-being. Try incorporating breathing exercises into your daily routine, such as alternate nostril breathing or lower diaphragmatic breathing.

③ **Pelvic Floor Exercises:** Strengthening the pelvic floor muscles can improve blood circulation in the reproductive organs, supporting their optimal functioning. Practice gentle pelvic floor exercises, such as Kegels, to enhance your sexual and reproductive health.

④ **Cultivating Sexual Energy:** Engage in conscious lovemaking with your partner, focusing on exchanging and harmonizing your Yin and Yang energies. Techniques such as eye gazing, synchronized breathing, and sensual touch can deepen your emotional and energetic connection, creating a fertile environment for conception.

⑤ **Nourish Your Body:** In TCM and Tantra, a healthy diet and lifestyle are crucial for maintaining optimal health and fertility. Consume nourishing, whole foods, and engage in gentle exercises such as yoga, tai chi, or qi gong to support your body's natural healing processes.

The practice of Tantra offers a holistic approach to fertility by nurturing the body, mind, and spirit. By integrating the principles of Tantra and Traditional Chinese Medicine, women over 40 can enhance their chances of conceiving.

The 4 Essentials of Tantra Sex Teachings:

Tantra is an ancient spiritual practice that transcends conventional ideas about sex and embraces sexual energy as a powerful force for spiritual growth, healing, and rejuvenation. By incorporating the four essentials of Tantra Sex Teachings – Conversation, Practice, Energy, and Purity – women over 40 can effectively improve your chances of conceiving and experience a deeper connection with your partner.

1. Conversation: The Pillar of Communication

Open, honest, and empathetic communication is at the heart of Tantra, and it is an essential element for couples trying to conceive. In Traditional Chinese Medicine, the concept of harmony between Yin and Yang is critical for maintaining balance in one's body and mind.

By engaging in a deep and meaningful conversation with your partner, you can create a harmonious environment that fosters trust, understanding, and emotional intimacy.

Discuss your intentions, desires, and concerns openly with your partner, and make sure to listen and respond with empathy. By doing so, you create a foundation of trust that allows for the free flow of energy (Qi) between you and your partner, thus enhancing your chances of conception.

2. Practice: Cultivating Sexual Energy

Tantra teaches that sexual energy is a potent life force that can be harnessed and transformed to nourish the body and spirit. In Traditional Chinese Medicine, this energy is known as Jing, which is believed to be the essence of life and fertility. As women age, their Jing naturally diminishes, which can make conception more challenging.

Tantric practices such as deep breathing, meditation, and the cultivation of sexual energy through slow, mindful lovemaking can help replenish and strengthen a woman's Jing. By focusing on pleasure, connection, and the exchange of energy, rather than a goal-oriented approach to sex, you can create an environment that nurtures fertility and promotes conception.

3. Energy: Balancing the Flow of Qi

Qi is the vital life force that flows through the body, and maintaining a balanced flow of Qi is essential for optimal health and fertility. In Traditional Chinese Medicine, imbalances in Qi can manifest as physical, emotional, or spiritual issues that may impact fertility.

Incorporating Tantra teachings into your daily life can help regulate the flow of Qi and support the body's natural ability to conceive.

Techniques such as conscious breathing, meditation, and self-massage can help to release blockages and stimulate the flow of energy throughout your body.

By focusing on your breath and the sensations in your body, you become more attuned to the subtle energies within, allowing for a deeper connection with your partner and a greater likelihood of conception.

4. Purity: A Holistic Approach to Mind, Body, and Spirit

Purity, in the context of Tantra, refers to a holistic approach to health and well-being that encompasses the mind, body, and spirit. From a Traditional Chinese Medicine perspective, purity is achieved through living in harmony with nature, nurturing one's physical health, and cultivating spiritual balance.

By integrating the four essentials of Tantra Sex Teachings into your life, you cansignificantly enhance your chances of conceiving. This holistic approach not only fosters a deeper connection with your partner but also empowers you to take charge of your fertility and overall well-being.

Conscious Creation: Calling in the Soul

Creating Scared Space for a Soul to Enter

As you work to cultivate your sexual energy and optimize your fertility through TCM practices, it's essential to create a sacred space for the soul you wish to call in. To do this:

① **Connect with your partner:** Engage in open and honest communication with your partner about your intentions, hopes, and dreams for your future family. This shared intention can strengthen your bond and create a welcoming environment for a soul to enter.

② **Cultivate love and gratitude:** Cultivating a loving and grateful mindset is essential for calling in a soul. Focus on the love and joy that you and your partner share, and envision the love you will give to your future child. Expressing gratitude for the life you have and the life you are creating can help to generate positive energy, which in turn supports fertility and attracts the soul you wish to bring into your family.

③ **Create a nurturing environment:** Make your home a sanctuary that reflects the love, peace, and tranquility you wish to share with your future child. Incorporate elements of nature, soft lighting, and soothing colors to create a space that feels warm and welcoming.

④ **Develop a spiritual practice:** Engaging in regular spiritual practices such as meditation, yoga, or prayer can help you connect with your inner wisdom and the divine source of creation. These practices can also help to reduce stress and promote emotional well-being, which are essential for fertility.

⑤ **Honor your body:** Treat your body as the sacred temple it is by engaging in regular self-care practices. This includes getting enough sleep, exercising regularly, and indulging in nurturing activities such as massages or warm baths. By honoring and respecting your body, you create a welcoming environment for a soul to enter.

Embracing the Journey and Trusting the Process

As you integrate Tantra and TCM into your life to enhance fertility, it's essential to be patient and trust in the process. Remember that every woman's journey is unique and that there is no set timeline for conception. By cultivating love, gratitude, and a nurturing environment, you are creating the optimal conditions for a soul to enter your life.

Stay open to the wisdom and guidance that both Tantra and TCM offer, and allow yourself to be guided by your intuition as you navigate your fertility journey. By focusing on the mind-body-spirit connection, you can create a powerful foundation for conscious creation and prepare yourself to host a soul in your loving and nurturing environment.

Combining the ancient wisdom of Tantra with the healing practices of Traditional Chinese Medicine can provide a transformative path for women over 40 who are seeking to conceive. By cultivating sexual energy, nourishing the body and mind, and creating a sacred space for a soul to enter, you are actively participating in the process of conscious creation and preparing yourself to host a soul with love, gratitude, and open-heartedness.

Myth: Tantra is Not Sex

Tantra: Beyond the Sexual Stereotype

When most people hear the term "Tantra," they often associate it with exotic sexual practices. While it's true that Tantra does address sexuality, it's essential to understand that it is much more than just sex. Tantra is an ancient spiritual practice that originated in India around 5,000 years ago. It is a holistic approach that combines yoga, meditation, and other practices to awaken and balance the body's energy centers, known as "chakras."

In the context of TCM, Tantra is a powerful tool to help cultivate and balance one's Qi. The study of Tantra is about harnessing and directing energy through the body, mind, and spirit to promote overall well-being, including fertility.

The Role of Energy in Fertility

According to TCM, a woman's fertility is deeply connected to the balance and flow of Qi in her body. When energy flows freely, it nourishes and supports the reproductive organs, allowing for optimal fertility.

On the other hand, when Qi becomes stagnant or blocked, it can lead to various health issues, including fertility challenges.

For women over 40 trying to conceive, maintaining a healthy energy balance is particularly crucial. As we age, our Qi naturally begins to decline, making it even more essential to focus on practices that can help rejuvenate and balance our energy levels.

Embracing the Mind–Body–Spirit Connection

As you delve deeper into Tantra, you'll discover the powerful connection between your mind, body, and spirit. Recognizing and embracing this connection is crucial for women over 40 trying to conceive. By nurturing all aspects of your being, you create a harmonious environment that supports your fertility journey.

① **Emotional well-being:** Emotional stress can have a significant impact on fertility. Make time to practice self-care and address any emotional issues that may be affecting your Ill-being.

This might include journaling, seeking therapy or counseling, or engaging in activities that bring joy and relaxation.

② **Spiritual Connection:** For many women, connecting with their spirituality can be a source of strength and support during their fertility journey. Engaging in practices such as prayer, mindfulness, or spending time in nature can help foster a deeper spiritual connection and promote inner peace.

③ **Physical Health:** Prioritizing physical health is essential for fertility. Maintain a healthy diet, exercise regularly, and get enough sleep to keep your body in optimal condition.

Building a Support Network

Navigating the fertility journey can be challenging, especially for women over 40. Building a support network of like-minded individuals, healthcare professionals, and TCM practitioners can provide invaluable guidance, encouragement, and resources. Consider joining local or online support groups focused on fertility, where you can share experiences, learn from others, and build connections with people who understand your journey.

Tantra offers a holistic approach to cultivating and balancing energy, which can be particularly beneficial for women over 40 trying to conceive. By incorporating Tantra practices into your daily routine and nurturing the mind-body-spirit connection, you can create a supportive environment for conception and overall well-being. Remember to listen to your body, seek support when needed, and embrace the power of your energy on your fertility journey.

What is Spiritual Sexuality and How to Use Energy During Lovemaking

Spiritual sexuality is the practice of engaging in sexual activities with the intention of connecting not only physically, but also emotionally and spiritually with your partner. This holistic approach to lovemaking involves a deep understanding of your own body, your partner's body, and the energies that flow between you.

It encourages mutual respect, trust, and intimacy, creating an ideal environment for conception, and harnessing and directing the flow of energy during lovemaking to improve fertility and conception chances.

Using Energy During Lovemaking: A TCM Perceptive

① **Cultivating Qi According to TCM.** The key to fertility lies in maintaining a healthy flow of Qi throughout the body. To cultivate your Qi, begin by incorporating breathing exercises and meditation into your daily routine. This will help you become more in tune with your body and its energies, which can be harnessed during lovemaking to enhance fertility.

② **Channeling Sexual Energy.** During sexual activity, focus on channeling your sexual energy through your body, directing it towards your reproductive organs. To do this, visualize warm, glowing energy emanating from your abdomen as you engage in deep, rhythmic breathing. This practice can help increase blood flow to your reproductive organs, improving their overall function and increasing the likelihood of conception.

③ **The Power of Intention.** Before engaging in sexual activity, set an intention with your partner to create a nurturing and supportive environment for conception. This can be done through open communication, discussing your desires, fears, and hopes, as well as any emotional or physical challenges you may be facing. By sharing your intentions, you create a strong bond with your partner, which can help alleviate stress and promote relaxation during lovemaking.

④ **Balancing Yin and Yang Energies.** In TCM, fertility is directly related to the balance of Yin (female) and Yang (male) energies within the body. When these energies are in harmony, the body is better equipped to support conception. To balance these energies during lovemaking, incorporate slow, gentle movements with more vigorous, passionate ones. This harmonious blend of energies will create a nurturing environment for conception and help facilitate the flow of Qi throughout your body.

⑤ **Cultivating a Spiritual Connection.** Finally, spiritual sexuality is about more than just physical pleasure; it's about connecting with your partner on a deeper level. To cultivate this connection, engage in activities that promote intimacy and trust, such as eye gazing, synchronized breathing, and gentle touch. These practices can help you and your partner feel more connected, both emotionally and energetically, creating a supportive environment for fertility.

The 7 Different Female Orgasms Explained

From the perspective of Traditional Chinese Medicine (TCM), sexual energy and the flow of Qi (vital energy) are interconnected, both playing crucial roles in fertility. For women over 40 seeking to conceive, understanding the various types of female orgasms can empower them to harness their sexual energy in order to improve their overall reproductive health. In this sub-chapter, I will delve into the seven different types of female orgasms and how they can be used in tandem with TCM principles to enhance fertility.

1. Clitoral Orgasm

One of the most well-known types of orgasms, the clitoral orgasm, is achieved through the stimulation of the clitoris, a highly sensitive area filled with nerve endings. In TCM, the clitoris is believed to be a powerful energy center that, when stimulated, can help enhance the flow of Qi and Blood throughout the body. For women trying to conceive, regular clitoral orgasms can support the health of the reproductive organs, ensuring a smoother path to conception.

2. Vaginal Orgasm

Vaginal orgasms are often described as deeper and more intense than clitoral orgasms. They occur through stimulation of the G-spot, located within the front wall of the vagina. According to TCM, the G-spot is a significant acupressure point that can help regulate menstrual cycles, balance hormones, and strengthen the uterus. Stimulating this area through sexual activity or self-massage can enhance the flow of Qi and blood to the reproductive organs, thereby increasing the chances of conception.

3. Blended Orgasm

A blended orgasm is a combination of clitoral and vaginal orgasms experienced simultaneously. This powerful orgasmic experience is known to release a surge of endorphins and oxytocin, which can help reduce stress and promote overall well-being. In TCM, blended orgasms can harmonize Yin and Yang energies, thereby increasing fertility potential in women over 40.

4. Cervical Orgasm

Cervical orgasms are achieved through deep penetration, which stimulates the cervix. In TCM, the cervix is considered to be the gateway to the uterus and an essential part of the female reproductive system. By gently massaging and stimulating the cervix during intercourse or self-massage, the flow of Qi and Blood can be increased, promoting the health of the reproductive organs and ultimately improving fertility.

5. Nipple Orgasm

The stimulation of the nipples can lead to an orgasm for some women. In TCM, the breasts and nipples are closely connected to the Heart and Liver meridians. Nipple orgasms can help open the Heart, allowing for a deeper connection with one's partner and promoting emotional healing. This release of emotional blockages can, in turn, improve fertility by enhancing the flow of Qi throughout the body.

6. Anal Orgasm

Although less common, anal orgasms can be experienced by women through the stimulation of nerve-rich areas surrounding the anus. In TCM, the anal area is linked to the Large Intestine meridian, which plays a role in the release of toxins from the body. Experiencing an anal orgasm can help eliminate blockages in the Large Intestine meridian, allowing for a more balanced flow of Qi and improved overall health, including increased fertility.

7. Energetic Orgasm

An energetic orgasm is a full-body experience that doesn't necessarily involve direct stimulation of the genitals. This type of orgasm can be achieved through practices like Tantra, deep breathing, or meditation. In TCM, energetic orgasms are believed to help balance the flow of Qi throughout the body and open up energy channels, promoting overall well-being and enhancing fertility potential. These orgasms also aid in the release of emotional and energetic blockages that may be inhibiting conception.

Connecting the 7 Orgarms to Fertility

Each of the seven female orgasms discussed in this sub-chapter plays a unique role in promoting fertility from the perspective of Traditional Chinese Medicine. Here are some tips on how to incorporate these orgasms into your journey to conception:

① **Mindful exploration:** Take time to discover your body's unique responses to different types of stimulation. By understanding your preferences, you can create an environment that facilitates the experience of multiple orgasms, fostering a harmonious flow of Qi and increasing your fertility potential.

② **Communicate with your partner:** Share your desires and preferences with your partner to create a supportive and nurturing sexual environment. This open communication will help you both experience deeper intimacy, enhancing the flow of Qi and improving your chances of conception.

③ **Practice Tantra:** Engage in Tantric practices with your partner or on your own. These practices, which often involve breathwork, meditation, and conscious movement, can help you cultivate energetic orgasms, balance your Qi, and create a fertile environment within your body.

④ **Incorporate TCM principles:** Complement your sexual exploration with other TCM practices, such as acupuncture, herbal remedies, and dietary changes. By addressing your overall health and well-being from a holistic perspective, you can further enhance your fertility potential.

⑤ **Prioritize self-care:** Emotional and physical well-being are closely linked to fertility. Prioritize self-care by engaging in stress-reduction techniques, exercise, and a nourishing diet to create a healthy foundation for conception.

Understanding the different types of female orgasms and their connection to fertility from a Traditional Chinese Medicine perspective can empower women over 40 seeking to conceive. By incorporating these orgasms into your sexual practice and balancing your Qi, you can create an optimal environment for conception and embark on a more fulfilling journey to motherhood. Remember that every woman's body is unique, and it is essential to listen to your body's needs and responses as you explore the rich landscape of female sexuality.

The Distinction between Orgasm and Ejaculation for Men

In the journey to fertility and conception, it is crucial for women over 40 to understand the subtleties and nuances of their partner's sexual health, particularly when it comes to male orgasm and ejaculation. From a Traditional Chinese Medicine (TCM) standpoint, the delicate balance of Yin and Yang energy is at play during the act of sexual intercourse. The mastery of this balance is the essence of Tantra, the ancient practice that transcends cultural and geographical boundaries.

In this sub-chapter, I will delve into the distinction between male orgasm and ejaculation from a TCM perspective, shedding light on how this knowledge can empower women over 40 who are trying to conceive. By understanding these concepts, couples can foster a deeper connection, enhance their sexual experiences, and ultimately improve their chances of conception.

Orgasm and Ejaculation: A Key Difference

At first glance, orgasm and ejaculation may appear to be synonymous. However, from a TCM and Tantric perspective, they are two distinct experiences that occur during sexual intercourse.

Orgasm is a culmination of pleasure, arousal, and sexual energy, often accompanied by involuntary muscle contractions and a release of tension. It is an experience that transcends the physical body and engages the emotional and spiritual aspects of a person. In TCM, an orgasm is a harmonious exchange of Yin and Yang energies, which can create a powerful connection between partners.

Ejaculation, on the other hand, is the physiological act of expelling semen from the male body. In TCM, semen is considered to contain a man's vital essence or Jing. The preservation of Jing is crucial to maintain overall health, strength, and vitality. While ejaculation is a natural part of the male sexual response, overindulgence in this act can lead to the depletion of vital energy and compromise a man's health, as well as his fertility potential.

Tantric Practices for Men: Harnessing Sexual Energy

In the practice of Tantra, men are encouraged to learn techniques that allow them to separate orgasm from ejaculation, thereby preserving their vital essence and enhancing their sexual experiences. By developing a deeper understanding of their own bodies and the flow of energy within them, men can learn to harness their sexual energy and channel it toward spiritual and emotional growth.

One technique that can be practiced by men is the art of non-ejaculatory orgasm, also known as "dry orgasm" or "valley orgasm." This practice involves the development of pelvic floor muscles and the mastery of breath control to help prevent ejaculation during orgasm. The result is a full-body experience that conserves vital energy, increases stamina, and strengthens the bond between partners.

How this Knowledge Benefits Women Over 40

As a woman in her 40s seeking to conceive, understanding the distinction between orgasm and ejaculation and the practices associated with Tantra can have a positive impact on your fertility journey. By encouraging your partner to explore and practice Tantric techniques, you can:

1. Foster a deeper emotional and spiritual connection with your partner, enhancing the overall quality of your relationship.

2. Increase your partner's sexual stamina and vitality, which may improve your chances of conception.

3. Preserve your partner's vital essence, supporting his overall health and fertility potential.

4. Encourage a more mindful approach to intimacy, creating an environment that is conducive to conception.

The art of Tantra, with its focus on the harmonious balance of Yin and Yang energies, offers a valuable perspective on the distinction between orgasm and ejaculation for men. By embracing these concepts and incorporating Tantric practices into your intimate life, you and your partner can experience a deeper connection, improve your overall well-being, and increase your chances of conception.

Semen Retention: Orgasm Control Practices and Techniques

The art of sexual ecstasy and tantra revolves around the balance and flow of energy within the body. Semen retention and orgasm control are powerful practices that can enhance fertility and overall well-being. By learning to control and channel this energy, you can improve your chances of conceiving and experiencing a deeper connection with your partner.

The Role of Kidney Essence and Jing

In TCM, the Kidney system plays a crucial role in fertility. The Kidney Essence, also known as Jing, is the basis for growth, development, and reproduction. As men age, the levels of Jing naturally decline, which may affect fertility. By practicing semen retention and orgasm control, you can conserve and even replenish your Jing, thereby improving your reproductive health.

The Concept of Yin and Yang

Yin and Yang are fundamental concepts in TCM, representing the dynamic balance between opposing forces in the universe. In the context of fertility and sexual energy, Yin represents the feminine, nurturing, and receptive aspects, while Yang represents the masculine, active, and penetrating aspects. A harmonious balance between Yin and Yang is essential for optimal fertility. Semen retention and orgasm control practices can help to maintain and restore this balance.

Techniques for Semen Retention and Orgasm Control

① **Deep Breathing and Meditation:** Cultivating a deep, relaxed breath helps to calm the mind and body, allowing for a greater connection with your inner self. This can help you become more aware of the sensations in your body, ultimately leading to better control over your sexual energy. Guided meditation practices focusing on fertility can also enhance your connection to your reproductive system and support your conception journey.

② **Pelvic Floor Exercises (Kegels):** Strengthening your pelvic floor muscles can improve your ability to control the flow of sexual energy within your body. Regular practice of Kegel exercises not only helps with orgasm control but also enhances sexual pleasure.

③ **Circulating Energy (Microcosmic Orbit):** In TCM, the Microcosmic Orbit is a vital energy channel that connects the body's main energy centers. By learning to circulate sexual energy through this channel, you can nurture your Kidney Essence and support your fertility. To practice this technique, visualize your sexual energy moving up your spine, over your head, and then down the front of your body, creating a continuous circuit.

④ **Non-Ejaculatory Orgasms:** By developing the ability to experience deep, full-body orgasms without the release of sexual fluids, you can conserve your Jing and maintain your Yin and Yang balance.

⑤ **Cultivating a Mindful and Loving Connection:** Fostering a deep, emotional connection with your partner is essential for a fulfilling sexual experience and a healthy conception. Approaching intimacy from a place of love, trust, and open communication can help you both develop greater control over your sexual energy and enhance your fertility.

Semen retention and orgasm control practices can offer significant benefits for both men and women who are trying to conceive. By cultivating a deeper connection with your body, your partner, and your sexual energy, you can support your reproductive health and overall well-being.

Tantra Sexual Practices for Conscious Conception

As a holistic approach, Tantra seeks to balance and harmonize the body, mind, and spirit. In this sub-chapter, I will explore how the art of Tantra, with its emphasis on sexual ecstasy, can be integrated with TCM to enhance fertility for women over 40. By engaging in the following practices, men and women can cultivate their sexual energy and improve their chances of conscious conception.

1. Soul Gazing

Soul gazing is a powerful tantric practice that fosters deep emotional intimacy and spiritual connection between partners. It involves sitting face-to-face, gazing into each other's eyes without any distractions, and allowing the energy to flow freely between you. This practice helps balance the Yin and Yang energies, which TCM believes are essential for conception.

For women over 40, soul gazing can help release emotional blockages and create a stronger connection with their partners. It can also increase the flow of Qi (life force energy) and Blood throughout the body, which is essential for reproductive health.

2. Tantric and Taoist Massage and Bodywork: Abdominal Massage, Sensual Erotic Massage

Abdominal massage and sensual erotic massage are two powerful techniques forcultivating sexual energy and enhancing fertility. In TCM, the abdomen is considered a vital energy center, housing organs responsible for reproduction, digestion, and elimination. By gently massaging the abdomen, you can help improve blood flow, release tension, and unblock stagnant Qi.

Sensual erotic massage, on the other hand, focuses on stimulating erogenous zones and awakening sexual energy. This practice is beneficial for women over 40 as it helps increase libido, improves circulation, and supports hormonal balance.

3. Genital Mapping

Genital mapping, also known as Yoni and Lingham mapping, is a transformative practice that encourages self-discovery and deepens the connection between partners. It involves gently exploring the genitals, both internally and externally, to uncover areas of tension, pleasure, and sensitivity.

For women over 40, yoni mapping can help identify and release any physical or emotional blockages that may be hindering fertility.

It can also help you connect more deeply with your womb, which is essential for creating a welcoming environment for conception.

Lingham mapping can help you and your partner understand their own body better and create a deeper connection between you. This shared understanding and intimacy can provide a strong foundation for conscious conception.

4. Womb Meditation and Practices for Womb Healing

Womb meditation is a practice that allows you to connect with the energy and wisdom of your womb. By focusing your attention on this sacred space, you can tap into your innate feminine power and enhance your fertility. This can be particularly beneficial for women over 40, as it encourages self-awareness and healing.

To begin a womb meditation, find a quiet, comfortable space where you can sit or lie down. Close your eyes, take a few deep breaths, and bring your awareness to your womb.
Visualize a warm, glowing light emanating from this area, and allow it to expand with each breath. As you connect with your womb,

you may experience emotions, memories, or sensations—welcome these experiences without judgment and let them flow through you.

In addition to meditation, other practices such as yoga, qigong, and breathwork can help you connect with your womb and improve your fertility. By incorporating these practices into your daily routine, you can create a nurturing environment for conception and enhance your overall Ill-being.

By engaging in these Tantra sexual practices and integrating them with the principles of Traditional Chinese Medicine, women over 40 can increase their chances of conscious conception. These practices not only cultivate sexual energy but also support emotional, physical, and spiritual well-being.

By working with a partner or on your own, you can develop a deeper understanding of your body, release blockages, and create an optimal environment for conception. For women in their 40s, this holistic approach to fertility is particularly important, as it addresses not only the physical aspects of reproduction but also the emotional and energetic components.

Through soul gazing, tantric and Taoist massage, genital mapping, and womb meditation, you can connect with your innate feminine power and enhance your fertility. These practices encourage self-awareness, emotional healing, and the free flow of Qi and Blood, which are essential for a healthy pregnancy.

Remember that the journey to conscious conception is unique for each individual. Be patient with yourself and your body, and honor the process as it unfolds. By embracing the art of Tantra and integrating it with Traditional Chinese Medicine, you can empower yourself and create the optimal conditions for bringing a new life into the world.

Made in the USA
Middletown, DE
05 November 2023

41941830R00186